THE
NERVOUS
SYSTEM

Second Edition

THE
NERVOUS SYSTEM
Introduction and Review

Charles R. Noback, Ph.D.
Professor of Anatomy
College of Physicians and Surgeons
Columbia University

Robert J. Demarest
Director, Medical Illustration
College of Physicians and Surgeons
Columbia University

McGraw-Hill Book Company
A Blakiston Publication

New York　　St. Louis　　San Francisco　　Auckland
Bogotá　　Düsseldorf　　Johannesburg　　London
Madrid　　Mexico　　Montreal　　New Delhi　　Panama
Paris　　São Paulo　　Singapore　　Sydney　　Tokyo　　Toronto

Library of Congress Cataloging in Publication Data

Noback, Charles Robert, date
    The nervous system.

    "A Blakiston publication."
    Includes index.
    1. Nervous system. I. Demarest, Robert J.,
joint author. II. Title. [DNLM: 1. Nervous
system—Anatomy & histology. 2. Neurophysiology.
WL101 N744n]
QP361.N6   1977   612'.8   76-46303
ISBN 0-07-046849-4

THE NERVOUS SYSTEM: Introduction and Review

1 2 3 4 5 6 7 8 9 0   DODO   7 8 3 2 1 0 9 8 7

This book was set in Times Roman by York Graphic Services, Inc.
The editors were J. Dereck Jeffers and Richard S. Laufer;
the cover was designed by Nicholas Krenitsky;
the production supervisor was Robert C. Pedersen.
R. R. Donnelley & Sons Company was printer and binder.

Contents

Preface

This second edition, retaining the basic organization of the first edition, presents a brief account of the basic elements of the human nervous system. The organization is designed and directed to meet the needs of two groups primarily: (1) the beginning student who wants an introductory yet reasonably comprehensive survey of this subject, and (2) the reader with background who wants to review rapidly the overall aspects and some pertinent details of this discipline.

The beginning student, it is hoped, will be able to get a firmer grasp sooner than otherwise of the basic and meaningful outlines of what at first appears to be a bewildering labyrinth of information. Readers who want to brush up and review can readily find those topics of immediate interest to them. Functional anatomicoclinical correlations are included primarily to point up those structural and physiologic aspects and are significant and relevant to an understanding of the nervous system. Some new illustrations and recent advances have been added to keep the book up-to-date.

We wish to extend our thanks to those students and colleagues who made valuable suggestions for improvement.

Charles R. Noback
Robert J. Demarest

THE
NERVOUS
SYSTEM

Introduction and Terminology

A baffling uncertainty is, to most students, the hallmark of the initial stages of a course in neuroanatomy. Not until many facets of the subject blend, in the latter half of the course, does a student feel a gain in control over the material. To ameliorate the uncertain feeling, the user of this book should read the text and examine the figures in the first four chapters (especially Chap. 1) for a general understanding only, then use them later for reference. A comprehension of Chaps. 5 through 10 is useful because this block contains (1) basic information relating to the concept of the pathway systems and (2) background knowledge for the remaining chapters in the book.

The nervous system and the endocrine system harmonize the many complex functional activities of the body. The former is the rapid coordinator, whereas the latter is more deliberate in its action.

DIVISIONS OF THE NERVOUS SYSTEM

The unpaired, bilaterally symmetric nervous system is subdivided (1) anatomically into the central nervous system and the peripheral nervous system, and (2) functionally into the somatic nervous system and the autonomic (visceral) nervous system.

The *central nervous system* (CNS) comprises the brain and spinal cord, which are encapsulated within the skull and vertebral column, respectively. The *peripheral nervous system* includes the cranial and spinal nerves associated, respectively, with the brain and spinal cord. The peripheral nerves convey (1) neural messages from the sense organs and sensory receptors in the organism as sensory input to the CNS and (2) neural impulses from the CNS as motor output to the muscles and glands of the body.

The *somatic nervous system* comprises those neural structures of the CNS involved with (1) conveying and processing conscious and unconscious sensory (afferent) information—e.g., vision, pain, touch, unconscious muscle sense—from the head, body wall, and extremities to the CNS, and (2) motor control of the voluntary (striated) muscles. The *autonomic nervous system* comprises those neural structures involved with (1) conveying and processing sensory input from the visceral organs (e.g., digestive system and cardiovascular system), and (2) motor activities influencing the involuntary (smooth) and cardiac musculature and glands of the viscera. Many authors consider the autonomic nervous system to be exclusively a visceral motor system (see Chap. 17).

Sensory signals originating in the sensory receptors are monitored by, processed in, and transmitted through the nervous system by systems known as *ascending sensory pathways* (*circuits* or *tract* systems), e.g., pain and temperature pathways and the visual pathway. These inputs may reach the conscious sphere or may be utilized at unconscious levels. The neural messages modulating and regulating motor activity are processed in and conveyed through the nervous system to the muscles and glands by systems known as *descending motor pathways*. Both the ascending sensory and descending motor pathways are hierarchically organized, with processing centers (e.g., ganglia, nuclei, laminae, cortex) for each pathway located at different anatomic levels of the spinal cord and brain. The processing centers are the computers of this immensely complex, high-speed system, which is undoubtedly more intricate than any made by humans.

From the sensory receptors in the body to the highest centers in the CNS, each *ascending sensory pathway system* follows, in a general way, a basic sequence: (1) Sensory receptors, e.g., touch corpuscles of Meissner in the skin, transmit by (2) nerve fibers, which convey signals to (3) processing centers in the spinal cord and brain, from which signals are conveyed by (4) other nerve fibers, which may ascend on the same side of the CNS or may cross over to (decussate) and ascend on the opposite side of the CNS before terminating in (5) higher processing centers; from these centers (6) other nerve fibers ascend on the same side before terminating in (7) the highest processing centers in the cerebral cortex. Differences in the basic sequence are present in some ascending systems.

In a general way, the *motor systems* are organized (1) to receive stimuli from the sensory systems at all levels of the spinal cord and brain, and (2) to convey messages via the descending motor pathways terminating in the head, body, and extremities to neuromuscular and neuroglandular endings at muscle and gland cells. The *descending motor pathways* comprise (1) sequences of processing centers and their fibers conveying neural influences to other processing centers within the CNS, and (2) the final linkages extending from the CNS via motor fibers of the peripheral nervous system to muscle and glands.

ORIENTATION IN THE BRAIN

The long axis through the brain and spinal cord is called the *neuraxis*. It takes the form of a T, the vertical part being a line passing through the entire spinal cord and brainstem (medulla, pons, and midbrain) and the horizontal part being a line extending from the frontal pole to the occipital pole of the cerebrum (Fig. 1.2). In essence, the cerebral long axis is oriented at right angles to the long axis of the brainstem–spinal cord. The bend in the axis occurs at the junction of the midbrain and the diencephalon (Chap. 1).

The term *rostral* ("toward the beak") means in the direction of the cerebrum. *Caudal* means in the direction of the coccygeal region. These terms are used in relation to the neuraxis, not the body. In this usage, the cerebrum is rostral to the brainstem and the frontal pole of the cerebrum is rostral to the diencephalon. *Coronal sections* are those cut at right angles to the neuraxis. A coronal section of the cerebrum is at right angles to a coronal section of the brainstem or spinal cord. *Horizontal sections* are those cut parallel to the neuraxis. Horizontal sections through the cerebrum are cut from the frontal pole to the occipital pole, parallel to a plane passing through both eyes. Horizontal sections through the brainstem and spinal cord are cut rostrocaudally parallel to the front and back of the neuraxis. A *sagittal section* is cut in a vertical plane along the midline; it divides the CNS into two symmetric right and left halves. Midsagittal is sometimes used for sagittal. Parasagittal sections, then, are also in the vertical plane but lateral to the midsagittal section.

Afferent (or *-petal*, as in centripetal) refers to bringing to or into a structure such as a nucleus; afferent is often used for *sensory*. *Efferent* (or *-fugal*, as in centrifugal) refers to going away from a structure such as a nucleus; efferent is often used for *motor*.

ORGANIZATION OF NEURONS IN THE BRAIN

Within the CNS groups or columns of cell bodies and dendrites of neurons are variously known as a *nucleus, ganglion, lamina, body, cortex,* or *center.* A *cortex* is a laminated complex of gray matter located on the surface of the brain. Three cortices are recognized: cerebral cortex, cerebellar cortex, and superior colliculus of midbrain. These structures form the gray matter, which is a complex of cell bodies, dendrites, portions of myelinated and unmyelinated nerve fibers, and glial cells.

Bundles of nerve fibers in the CNS which are characterized by anatomic or functional criteria are called by such terms as *tract, fasciculus, brachium, peduncle, column, lemniscus, commissure, ansa,* or *capsule.* A *commissure* is a bundle of fibers crossing the midline at right angles to the neuraxis, often interconnecting similar structures on each side. A *decussation* refers to fibers crossing the midline either at right angles or obliquely. These structures are white matter, which is made up of myelinated and unmyelinated fibers and glial cells.

Contralateral refers to the opposite side; it is used primarily to indicate, for example, that pain is lost or paralysis occurs on the side opposite to that of the lesion. *Ipsilateral* refers to the same side; it is used primarily to indicate, for example, that pain is lost or paralysis occurs on the same side as that of the lesion.

A *modality* refers to the quality of a stimulus and the resulting forms of sensation (e.g., touch, pain, sounds, vision). Some pathways (tracts, nuclei, or areas of cortex) are *somatotopically* (*topographically*) organized; specific portions of these structures are associated with restricted regions of the body. For example, (1) fibers conveying position sense from the hand are in definite locations within the posterior columns (ascending sensory pathway), and (2) certain areas of the motor cortex regulate movements of the thumb. Some structures of the visual pathway are topographically related to specific regions within the retina (retinotopic organization), and similarly some structures of the auditory pathways are organized functionally with respect to different frequencies or tones (tonotopic organization).

Chapter 1

Gross Anatomy of the Brain

The average adult human brain weighs about 1,400 g, approximately 2 percent of the total body weight. The gelatinous brain is invested by a succession of three connective tissue membranes called *meninges* and is protected by an outer rigid capsule, the bony skull. The brain floats in cerebrospinal fluid, which supports it and acts as a shock absorber in rapid movements of the head. The major arteries and veins supplying the brain lie among the meninges.

SUBDIVISIONS OF THE BRAIN

The brain (encephalon) comprises five major subdivisions (Figs. 1.1 to 1.4): telencephalon, diencephalon, mesencephalon (midbrain), metencephalon, and myelencephalon (medulla oblongata, or medulla). The metencephalon, exclusive of the cerebellum, is called the *pons*. The telencephalon consists of two *cerebral hemispheres*).

The *cerebrum* includes the telencephalon and diencephalon. The *brain-stem* comprises the diencephalon (some classifications exclude this), mesen-

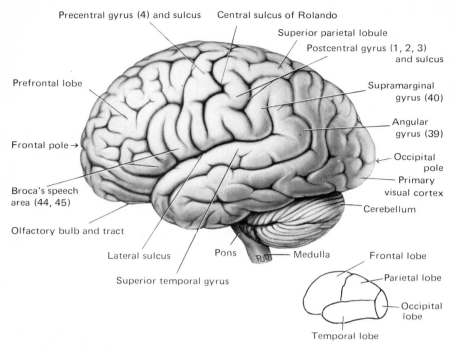

Figure 1.1 Lateral surface of the brain. Numbers refer to Brodmann's areas.

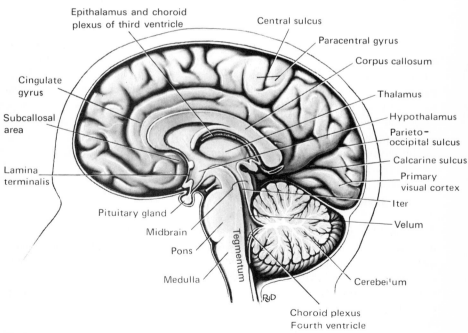

Figure 1.2 Median sagittal section of the brain.

6

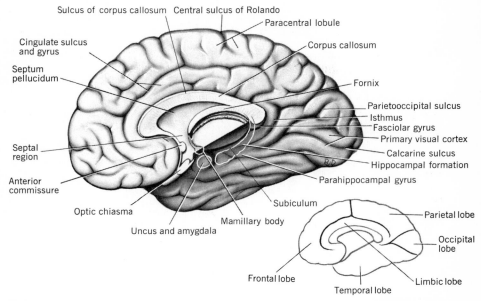

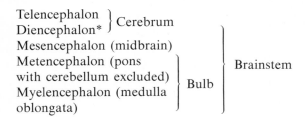

Figure 1.3 Median surface of the cerebral hemisphere. The amygdaloid body and hippocampal formation are represented by white lines. The subcortical amygdaloid body is located within the uncus. The hippocampal formation (hippocampus and dentate gyrus) is located in the floor of the temporal horn of the lateral ventricle (see Fig. 1.4).

cephalon, pons, and medulla. The lower brainstem—pons and medulla—is called the *bulb* (bulbar region). These subdivisions of the encephalon are outlined as follows:

$$
\left.
\begin{array}{l}
\left.\begin{array}{l}\text{Telencephalon}\\ \text{Diencephalon*}\end{array}\right\}\text{Cerebrum}\\
\text{Mesencephalon (midbrain)}\\
\left.\begin{array}{l}\text{Metencephalon (pons}\\ \text{with cerebellum excluded)}\\ \text{Myelencephalon (medulla}\\ \text{oblongata)}\end{array}\right\}\text{Bulb}
\end{array}
\right\}\text{Brainstem}
$$

The brainstem is subdivided by its topographic relation to the dural structure called the tentorium (Fig. 4.1) into the *supratentorial* and *infratentorial divisions*. The diencephalon is the supratentorial division, and the midbrain, pons, and medulla make up the infratentorial division. All cranial nerves except the olfactory and optic nerves emerge from the infratentorial brainstem.

*Sometimes considered a part of the brainstem.

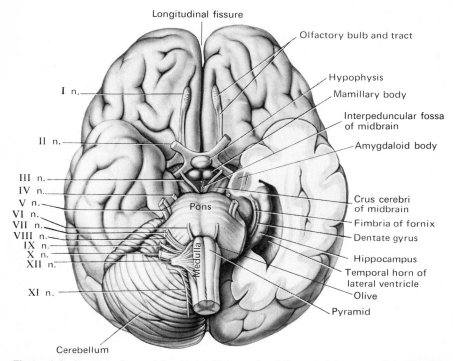

Figure 1.4 Basal surface of the brain. Note roots of the cranial nerves. A horizontal section has been made through the right temporal and occipital lobes; note the hippocampus, dentate gyrus, fornix, and temporal horn of the lateral ventricle. The hypophysis and the mamillary body are included in the diencephalon. n, cranial nerve.

The ventricular system (Chap. 4) is a continuous series of cavities within the brain filled with cerebrospinal fluid (Figs. 1.5 and 4.2). It is subdivided as follows: the paired *lateral ventricles* are the cavities of the telencephalon; the median *third ventricle* is within the diencephalon; the tubelike *cerebral aqueduct of Sylvius* (or *iter*) is the midbrain portion; and the *fourth ventricle* is within the metencephalon and medulla (Fig. 1.2).

CEREBRUM

The *cerebrum* comprises the two cerebral hemispheres and the diencephalon, which lies deep to the hemispheres. Each hemisphere is covered by a cortex of gray matter. White matter, basal ganglia (large nuclei), and the corpus callosum lie deep to the gray matter. The *corpus callosum* is a massive bundle of nerve fibers which interconnects the cortices of the two hemispheres.

Cerebral Topography

The hemispheres are marked by slitlike incisures called *sulci*. The raised ridges between sulci are *gyri*. The hemispheres are separated from one another in the midline by the *longitudinal fissure*. Each hemisphere is conventionally divided into six *lobes:* frontal, parietal, occipital, temporal, central (insula, or island of Reil), and limbic.

Lobes   The lobes are delineated from each other by several major sulci including the lateral sulcus of Sylvius, central sulcus of Rolando, cingulate sulcus, and parieto-occipital sulcus. The lateral sulcus is a deep furrow which extends posteriorly from the basal surface of the brain along the lateral surface of the hemisphere, to terminate usually as an upward curve between the angular gyrus and the supramarginal gyrus of the parietal lobe (Fig. 1.1). The central sulcus of Rolando extends obliquely from the region of the lateral sulcus across the dorsolateral cerebral surface and for a short distance onto the medial surface (Fig. 1.3). The cingulate sulcus is a curved cleft on the medial surface extending parallel to the curvature of the corpus callosum. The parieto-occipital sulcus is a deep cleft on the medial surface located between the central sulcus and the occipital pole.

The boundaries of the lobes on the lateral cerebral surface are as follows: (1) The frontal lobe is located anterior to the central sulcus and above the lateral sulcus; (2) the parietal lobe is located posterior to the central sulcus, anterior to an imaginary parieto-occipital line (parallel to the parieto-occipital sulcus), and above the lateral sulcus and its imaginary posterior continuation toward the occipital pole; (3) the temporal lobe is located below the lateral sulcus and anterior to the imaginary parieto-occipital line; and (4) the occipital lobe is posterior to the imaginary parieto-occipital line. The *central lobe* is located at the bottom of the lateral sulcus of Sylvius, which is actually a deep fossa.

The boundaries of the lobes on the medial cerebral surface are as follows: (1) The frontal lobe is located rostral to a line formed by the central sulcus and the cingulate sulcus; (2) the parietal lobe is bounded by the central sulcus, cingulate sulcus, and parieto-occipital sulcus; (3) the temporal lobe is located lateral to the parahippocampal gyrus; (4) the occipital lobe is posterior to the parieto-occipital lobe; and (5) the limbic lobe is located central to the curved line formed by the cingulate sulcus and the collateral sulcus (the latter is located lateral to the parahippocampal gyrus). The limbic lobe is the ring of gyri bordered by this line; it includes the subcallosal area, cingulate gyrus, parahippocampal gyrus, hippocampus, dentate gyrus, and uncus.

Gyri   The *precentral gyrus* is anterior and parallel to the central sulcus of Rolando. The *postcentral gyrus* is posterior and parallel to the central sulcus.

The *paracentral lobule,* on the medial surface, is continuous with the precentral and postcentral gyri on the lateral surface and is partially divided by the central sulcus.

The cortex anterior to the central sulcus is motor in function; that posterior to the central sulcus is sensory in function. The postcentral gyrus and the posterior part of the paracentral gyrus are known as Brodmann areas 1, 2, and 3 (see Fig. 21.1) of the cerebral cortex. The precentral gyrus and anterior portion of the paracentral gyrus are called area 4 or the motor cortex. The *transverse gyri of Heschl* located in the upper part of the temporal lobe facing the lateral sulcus make up the primary receptive area for audition (areas 41 and 42). The cortex on either side of the calcarine sulcus is the primary receptive area for vision (area 17). The areas outside the primary receptive areas are called *association areas* (Chap. 22): Broca's area (Fig. 1.1), for example, is a cortical area (44, 45) associated with the formulation of speech. The functional aspects of the Brodmann areas are discussed in Chap. 22.

Basal Ganglia

The term *basal ganglia* refers to several masses of subcortical nuclei deep in the cerebral hemispheres (Fig. 1.5). They include the caudate nucleus and lenticular nucleus, amygdaloid body (amygdala), and the claustrum (strip of detached cortex of central lobe). The *lenticular and caudate nuclei* are collectively called the *corpus striatum.* The *lenticular (lentiform) nucleus* is divided into the medially located globus pallidus (pallidum, paleostriatum) and the laterally located putamen. The putamen and the caudate nucleus are called the *striatum (neostriatum).* The subthalamic nucleus and substantia nigra are often classified as basal ganglia (see also Chap. 21):

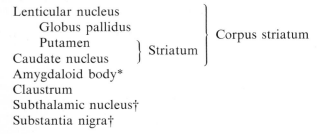

Diencephalon

The *diencephalon,* located in the ventromedial portion of the cerebrum, is continuous caudally with the midbrain (Fig. 1.2). It consists of four subdivisions: epithalamus, thalamus (dorsal thalamus), hypothalamus, and ventral

*Sometimes excluded.
†Sometimes included.

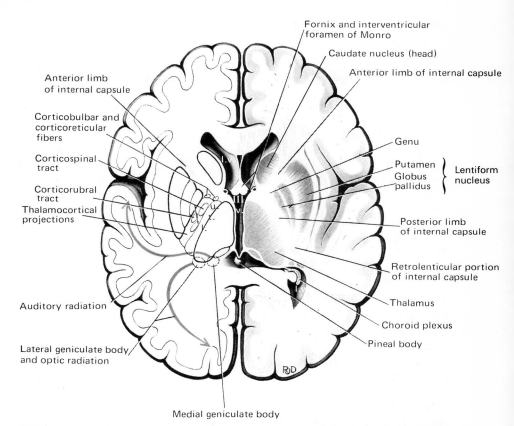

Fornix and interventricular foramen of Monro

Caudate nucleus (head)

Anterior limb of internal capsule

Anterior limb of internal capsule

Corticobulbar and corticoreticular fibers

Corticospinal tract

Corticorubral tract

Thalamocortical projections

Genu

Putamen
Globus pallidus
} Lentiform nucleus

Posterior limb of internal capsule

Retrolenticular portion of internal capsule

Auditory radiation

Thalamus

Choroid plexus

Pineal body

Lateral geniculate body and optic radiation

RJD

Medial geniculate body

Figure 1.5 Horizontal section through the cerebrum. Note the location of the head of the caudate nucleus, lenticular nucleus, thalamus relative to the ventricles and the internal capsule. The components of the internal capsule are indicated on the left side. U, upper extremity; T, trunk; L, lower extremity. Note that right lateral ventricle (lv.) is represented twice and the third ventricle (lllv.) once.

thalamus (subthalamus). The *epithalamus* is a narrow band of tissue in the region to which the choroid plexus of the third ventricle is attached; it includes the habenular nucleus and pineal body (see Chap. 19). The large *thalamus* is located dorsal to the hypothalamic sulcus (Chap. 20). Ventral to the hypothalamic sulcus are the *hypothalamus* and *hypophysis* or *pituitary gland* (Chap. 18). Lateral to the hypothalamus is the *subthalamus* (Chap. 21).

The *mamillary bodies* are located in the posterior hypothalamus. The optic nerves from the eye join as the *optic chiasma,* located anterior to the hypophysis, and continue caudally as the optic tracts, before terminating in the lateral geniculate bodies (nuclei) of the thalamus and superior colliculi of the midbrain (Chap. 16).

Internal Capsule (See Chap. 20)

The *internal capsule* is a massive bundle of nerve fibers which comprises almost all the fibers projecting from subcortical nuclei to the cerebral cortex or from the cerebral cortex to subcortical structures in the cerebrum, brainstem, and spinal cord (Figs. 11.2 and 11.3). It is divided into an anterior limb, genu, posterior limb, and a postlenticular (retrolenticular) part (Figs. 1.5 and 20.2). The *anterior (caudatolenticular) limb* is located between the head of the caudate nucleus and the lenticular nucleus. The *genu* (knee) is located between the anterior and posterior limbs. The *posterior (thalamolenticular) limb* is located between the lenticular nucleus and the thalamus. The *retrolenticular (postlenticular) part* of the posterior limb is located lateral to the thalamus and posterior to the lenticular nucleus.

BRAINSTEM—MIDBRAIN, PONS, AND MEDULLA

Anterior (Basal) Aspect

Several prominent landmarks are present on the anterior surface of the brainstem (Figs. 1.4 and 11.2). In the midbrain, the crura cerebri are lateral to the interpeduncular fossa through which passes the *oculomotor nerves* (*third cranial nerve*). The *trigeminal nerve* (*fifth cranial nerve*, composed of a small motor root and a large sensory root) emerges on the lateral aspect of the massive pons. The pyramids, olives, and roots of seven cranial nerves are features visible on the anterior surface of the medulla. The *pyramids* are formed by the fibers of the pyramidal tracts (corticospinal tract) which cross the midline at the pyramidal decussation in the lower medulla. The *olive* is a protuberance formed by the inferior olivary nucleus (Fig. 11.4D). From medial to lateral, the *abducent* (*sixth*), *facial* (*seventh*), and *vestibulocochlear* (*eighth*) *nerves* emerge at the pontomedullary junction. The *glossopharyngeal* (*ninth*) and *vagus* (*tenth*) *nerves* emerge as a series of rootlets from the postolivary sulcus on the posterior margin of the olive. The *spinal accessory* (*eleventh*) *nerve* emerges in the form of rootlets from the medulla (postolivary sulcus) and from the spinal cord (between the dorsal and ventral roots of the first six cervical spinal nerves). The *hypoglossal* (*twelfth*) *nerve* emerges from the preolivary sulcus between the olive and pyramid.

Note that the third, sixth, and twelfth cranial nerves emerge from the anterior brainstem in a longitudinal line just lateral to the midsagittal plane. The fifth, seventh, ninth, tenth, and eleventh cranial nerves emerge from the lateral aspect of the brainstem.

Posterior Aspect

The prominent landmarks on the posterior surface of the midbrain include the *superior colliculus* (optic system), *inferior colliculus* (auditory system), and *trochlear* (*fourth*) *nerve* (Figs. 11.1 and 11.2). The pontine and medullary structures viewed include the three *cerebellar peduncles* (*superior, middle, and inferior*) and some landmarks on the floor of the fourth ventricle. The floor is marked by a groove, the *sulcus limitans*. Medial to this groove are located the trigonum vagi and trigonum hypoglossi, and lateral to it is the area vestibularis. The *trigonum hypoglossi* is a short ridge formed by the underlying hypoglossal nucleus (Figs. 11.2 and 12.2). The *trigonum vagi* is formed by the underlying motor (parasympathetic) nucleus of the vagus nerve. The *area vestibularis* is the region of the vestibular nuclei. The *facial* (or *abducent*) *colliculus* is a hillock by the genu of the facial nerve and nucleus of the abducent nerve. On the dorsal surface of the inferior medulla are the *tuberculum gracilis* and *tuberculum cuneatus* formed by the nuclei gracilis and cuneatus, respectively. Note the diamond-shaped fourth ventricle (rhomboid fossa): the lateral recesses of the fourth ventricle lie at the level of the upper medulla. The roof of the fourth ventricle is *choroid plexus* (structure formed by the pia mater and its blood vessels in contact with ependyma lining the ventricle, Fig. 4.2).

Basilar Portion and Tegmentum of Brainstem

Anterior to the cerebral aqueduct of the midbrain and the fourth ventricle of the pons and medulla (Fig. 4.2), the brainstem consists of the tegmentum (adjacent to ventricle) and the basilar portion (on anterior aspect). The *basilar portion* comprises the *crura cerebri* of the midbrain cerebral peduncle, *pons proper* in the pons, and *pyramids* in the medulla (Figs. 11.2 and 11.3). The tracts within the basilar portion consist of the corticopontine fibers (terminate in pontine nuclei of pons proper), corticospinal tract, and some corticobulbar fibers. The bulk of the brainstem is the *tegmental portion* consisting of many nuclei and ascending and descending pathways. The pons consists of a *pons proper* (the *basilar portion*) and the *tegmental portion* of the pons.

The cerebral peduncle makes up one-half of the midbrain excluding the tectum. Each peduncle is divided into a tegmental (dorsal) part and a crus cerebri (ventral) part. The two are separated by gray matter called the *substantia nigra* (Fig. 11.5H).

Chapter 2

Neurons and Associated Cells

The neuron is the morphologic and functional unit of the nervous system. Each neuron is in contact (*synapse*) through its processes with other neurons, so that each is an interconnecting segment in the network composing the nervous system. Functionally each neuron is designed to react to stimuli, to transmit the resulting excitation rapidly to other portions of the cell, and to influence other neurons, muscle cells, and glandular cells. Neurons are so specialized that they are incapable of reproducing themselves, and they lose their viability if denied an oxygen supply for but several minutes.

Neurons exhibit a wide diversity of forms and sizes. With the exception of a few specialized types, each neuron usually consists of a *cell body* (also called *soma* or *nerve cell*) from which extends a single process called the *axon* and a variable number of branching processes called *dendrites* (*dendrons*). Each axon, or its collateral branches, terminates by arborizing into several filaments called *telodendria;* in turn, each telodendron ends with an enlargement called a *bouton terminal,* which is a part of a synaptic junction. At the other end of the neuron, the three-dimensional region through which the dendrites of a single nerve arborize is called its *dendritic field.*

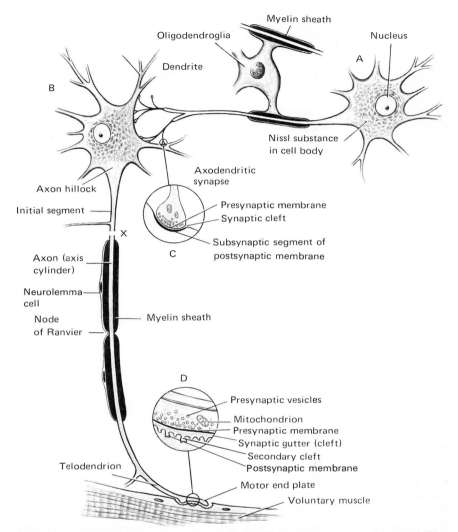

Figure 2.1 Diagram of (A) a neuron located within the central nervous system and (B) a lower motor neuron located in both the central and peripheral nervous systems. The latter synapses with a voluntary muscle cell to form a motor end-plate. Note the similarities, as reconstructed from electron micrographs, between (C) a synapse between two neurons and (D) a motor end-plate. The hiatus in the nerve at X represents the border between the central nervous system (above the X) and the peripheral nervous system (below the X).

ANATOMIC CONSIDERATIONS (Fig. 2.1)

The cell body contains a large nucleus, Nissl bodies, mitochondria and Golgi apparatus, and other inclusions. The nucleus has the same quantity of DNA as the nuclei in other cells; its prominent nucleolus, composed of RNA, is associated with synthesis of proteins. Within the nucleus are the sex chromatin bodies called nucleolar satellites, which are present in the female and absent in the male. The *Nissl bodies* are masses of granular (rough) endoplasmic reticulum with ribosomes, which are the protein-synthesizing machinery of the neuron. The prodigious amount of protein synthesized each day by a neuron, equal to about one-third of the protein in the cell body, is distributed by *axoplasmic flow* of neuroplasm down the axon. The *mitochondria,* which are numerous in the cell body, in the vicinity of the synapses, and in the nodes of Ranvier (see below), and the Golgi apparatus have the same functional roles as in somatic cells.

The dendrites contain the same cytoplasmic organelles (e.g., Nissl substance and mitochondria) that are present in the cell body; dendrites are true extensions of the cell body. Functionally the dendrite–cell body complex is the receptive and integrative unit of the neuron.

The axon (also called the *axis cylinder*) arises from the axon hillock of the cell body, at a site called the *initial segment,* and extends as a process from a fraction of a millimeter to as much as 1 m in length before branching into telodendria. The axon hillock, initial segment, and the axon lack Nissl substance. Each telodendron terminates as a bouton with a dendrite–cell body complex to form a synapse. The axon is an evolutionary specialization within a neuron for the transmission of coded information (as all-or-none action potentials) from the dendrite–cell body complex to the synaptic junctions.

Synapse

The *synapse* is the site of contact of one neuron with another (Figs. 2.1 and 2.2). A submicroscopic space, the synaptic cleft, which is about 200 Å exists between the bouton of one neuron and the cell body of another neuron (an *axosomatic synapse*), between the bouton of one neuron and a dendrite of another neuron (an *axodendritic synapse*), and between the bouton of one and an axon of another neuron (an *axoaxonic synapse*). *Dendrodendritic synapses* between two dendrites have been noted (e.g., in olfactory bulb and retina). The axon of one neuron may terminate in only a few synapses, or in many thousands of synapses. The dendrite–cell body complex may receive synaptic contacts from many different neurons (up to and over 15,000 synapses). The termination of a nerve fiber in a muscle cell (neuromuscular junction) or a glandular cell (neuroglandular junction) is basically similar to the synapse between two neurons. The synapse of each axon terminal of a motor neuron on a voluntary muscle cell is called a *motor end-plate.*

The cell membrane of the axon at the synapse is the *presynaptic membrane,* and the cell membrane of dendrite–cell body complex, muscle, or glandular cell is the *postsynaptic membrane.* The *subsynaptic membrane* is that region of the postsynaptic membrane (of the postsynaptic cell) that is juxtaposed against the presynaptic membrane at the synapse. A concentra-

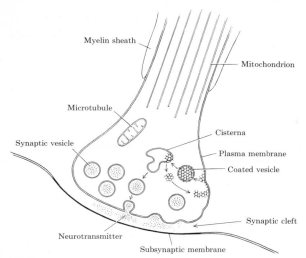

Figure 2.2 Neurotransmitters are synthesized in a neuron, stored and packaged in vesicles, and released by exocytosis. The transmitters and vesicles are recycled. Following exocytosis, the vesicle membrane fuses with the plasma membrane. New vesicle membranes are reformed by pinocytosis (endocytosis) from the plasma membrane and its intermediary structures, called cisternae. The coat of the newly formed vesicle is also recycled. (*After Heuser and Reese.*)

tion of mitochondria and small spherical vesicles called *presynaptic vesicles* (from 200 to 600 Å in diameter) is present in the cytoplasm of the bouton; no such concentration is present in the cytoplasm adjacent to the subsynaptic membrane. The vesicles contain the precursors of the active neurotransmitter agents (see below).

Peripheral Nervous System and Associated Cells

A peripheral nerve is composed of many nerve fibers, each of which is composed of an axon (axis cylinder), its neurolemma sheath, and a connective tissue (endoneural) sheath. The cells of the *neurolemma sheath* (*Schwann cells*) may elaborate a myelin sheath, a structure composed of concentric layers of the plasma membrane of these cells. A nerve fiber with a myelin sheath is said to be *myelinated,* and one with no myelin is *unmyelinated.* The myelin sheath is a segmented discontinuous layer, interrupted at regular intervals by the *nodes of Ranvier.* The distance from one node to the next is an *internode,* whose length is roughly proportional to the diameter of the fiber; the thicker the fiber, the longer its internodes. The diameters and lengths of internodes of the various fibers are directly related to the speed of conduction of the nerve impulse. Each internode is formed by and surrounded by one neurolemma (Schwann) cell. Three features of the nodes are important: (1) Nerve fibers branch at a node, (2) concentrations of mitochondria in the axis cylinder at these sites suggest a local high metabolic activity, and (3) the close proximity of extracellular fluids to the axon at each node is critical to saltatory conduction (see below). Nerve fibers are bound into *fascicles* by connective tissue.

CNS and Associated Cells (Neuroglia)

The neuroglia (*glia*) cells of the CNS outnumber its neurons 5 to 10 times and compose about 40 percent of the total volume of the brain and spinal cord.

The *oligodendroglia* (*oligodendrocytes*) are the equivalent to the neurolemma cells of the peripheral nerves (Fig. 2.1). The myelin sheaths of the axons in the CNS are products of the oligodendroglia, with each of these glial cells forming and maintaining the myelin sheaths (internodes) of several axons.

The *astroglia* (*astrocytes*) have numerous sheetlike processes extending from their cell bodies among the neurons (Fig. 2.3). These processes extend to (1) the basement lamina of the blood capillaries and form vascular feet, and (2) the piaglial membrane adjacent to the subarachnoid space at the surface of the brain. These glial cells have been implicated in providing essential nutrients for neurons, in the blood-brain barrier concept, in information storage processes, and in the maintenance of bioelectric potentials.

The *ependymal cells* are the glial cells which line the ventricular system and the choroid plexuses. They are involved in the production of cerebrospinal fluid.

The *microglia* are phagocytic cells which are related to the macrophages of the connective tissues. The microglia are found in small numbers throughout the CNS; under proper stress, as in an injury, they function to phagocytize and remove disintegration products of the neurons.

PHYSIOLOGIC CONSIDERATIONS

Each neuron is said to possess "in miniature the integrative capacity of the entire nervous system." The *dendrite–cell body unit* in most neurons is specialized as a receptor and integrator of synaptic input from other neurons, while the axon is specialized to convey coded information from the dendrite–cell body unit to the synaptic junctions, where transformation functions take place with other neurons or effectors (muscles and glands).

Information about the external world and the organism's internal environment is conveyed to the CNS via neurons of the peripheral nervous system called *first-order neurons*. The peripheral processes of these neurons terminate in the retina, cochlea, vestibular end organs, skin, muscles, joints, and internal viscera (e.g., stomach), while their central processes terminate with the CNS. The structural and functional features of a typical first-order neuron are described at the end of this chapter.

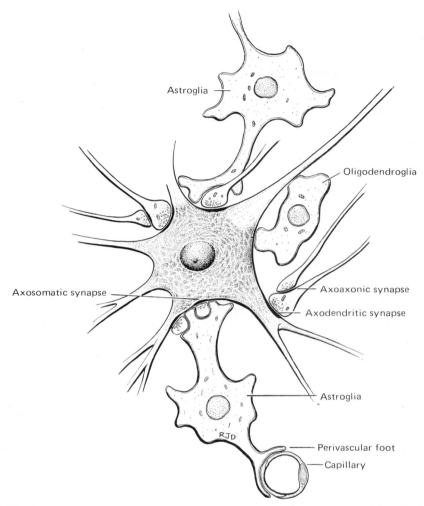

Figure 2.3 Relation of a neuron, astroglia, oligodendroglia, and nerve terminals. Note axosomatic synapse, axodendritic synapse, and axoaxonic synapse. Astroglia have processes extending to a capillary and to neurons.

Resting Membrane Potential

The *resting neuron* is a charged cell that is not conducting an impulse. The *cell* (*plasma*) *membrane* of the neuron acts as a thin boundary (50 to 100 Å thick) between two fluids—the interstitial (extracellular) fluid outside the neuron and the intracellular fluid (neuroplasm) inside the neuron (Fig. 2.4). Sodium (Na^+) and chloride (Cl^-) ions are in higher concentration in the

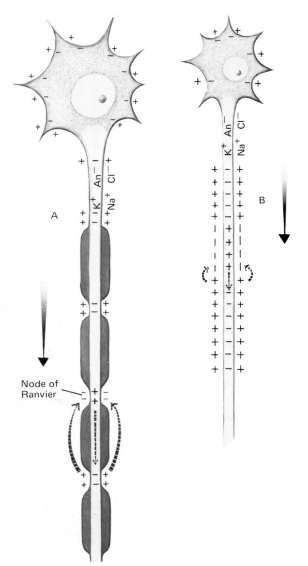

Figure 2.4 (A) A neuron with a myelinated axon and (B) a neuron with an unmyelinated axon showing the charges on the cell membrane and the location of certain ions in each neuron "at rest" and at active sites (one in each neuron) during conduction of an all-or-none action potential. The minus (−) sign within the neuron signifies an intraneuronal negativity with respect to the positivity (+) within the extracellular fluid outside the neuron. The two large arrows indicate the direction in which the nerve impulses are propagated. The interrupted arrows indicate the direction of the flow of current. Sodium, Na⁺; potassium, K⁺; chloride, Cl⁻; and protein, An⁻ ions.

interstitial fluid; potassium (K$^+$) and protein (organic) ions are in higher concentration in the intracellular fluid. As a result of the unequal distribution of ions across the semipermeable and selectively permeable cell membrane, the potential across the resting cell membrane is about -60 to -70 mV (with the excess of negative charge inside the cell). These differential concentrations of sodium (Na$^+$) ions and potassium (K$^+$) ions are produced and maintained by metabolic activity of the neuron (oxidative metabolism, ATP, and active transport); simultaneously the Na$^+$, which leaks into the neuron, is pumped out of the cell, and the K$^+$, which diffuses out, is pumped back into the neuron. This active process results in a concentration of K$^+$ within the neuroplasm which is 10 or more times higher than that within the interstitial (extracellular) fluid, and in concentrations of Na$^+$ and Cl$^-$, which are 10 times lower than those within the interstitial fluid.

Action Potential (All-or-None Activity, Nondecremental Conduction)

A variety of stimuli can alter the permeability of the cell membrane to certain ions and, in turn, bring about changes in the membrane potential. If a stimulus applied to an axon lowers the resting membrane potential to a critical voltage level, usually by 10 to 15 mV to the level of -30 to -50 mV, an explosionlike action results with the production of a brief electric phenomenon called an *action potential* (*spike, nerve impulse, all-or-none activity*). The action potential is the expression of a sudden reversal, known as *depolarization* of the Na$^+$/K$^+$ selectivity of the cell membrane of the axon, in which for a few milliseconds a polarity reversal occurs from the resting potential (-60 to -70 mV) to the action potential ($+30$ mV, with an excess of negative charge outside the neuron). The nerve fiber gains Na$^+$ and loses K$^+$ during the passage of the action potential.

The nerve impulse is propagated without decrement along all parts of the cell membrane of the axon as a continuous spread. Each depolarized patch on the membrane produces a flow of current (action potential), which sets off events to depolarize the adjacent patch, which, in turn, depolarizes the resting-charged region farther ahead. The action potential travels along the cell membrane as a chain reaction and regenerates itself from point to point along the axon without loss of amplitude and at a constant speed for that axon.

The axon possesses the energy for the action potential; the stimulus merely lowers the membrane potential sufficiently to trigger the axon into action. The axon gives an all-or-none, *on-off* response. The resting potential is restored within a millisecond or so after the action potential has passed by a site on the cell membrane. This smooth, progressive movement of the action potential is the presumed method of conduction in unmyelinated nerves (Fig. 2.4).

Saltatory Conduction

The action potential in a myelinated nerve is propagated by discontinuous spread or *saltatory (hop or jump) conduction*, in which the nerve impulse (depolarization) hops along the nerve fiber from node of Ranvier to node of Ranvier (Fig. 2.4). The current spreads from an active node to the next, inactive node. The nodes with their low thresholds are linked together by myelinated internodes (segmented insulating jackets) that act as passive conductors. Myelinated fibers are fast conductors of the action potentials. The speed of conduction of an action potential is related to the thickness of the myelin sheath and the lengths of the internodes of a nerve fiber. The thicker the myelin and the longer the internodes of a fiber, the faster the fiber conducts an action potential. The myelin improves the signaling efficiency of the axon.

Synapse

Of prime significance in the integrative activities of the nervous system is the synapse, which acts as a one-way valve, permitting the action potential of an axon to exert its influence across the synaptic cleft on the dendrite–cell body region (Fig. 2.1). Communication between neurons is through *neurotransmitters* (chemical agents), which are released at the nerve terminal (bouton) into the synaptic cleft, where they can influence the excitability of the postsynaptic neuron. The depolarization of the terminal by the action potential results in the influx of calcium (Ca^{++}) ions across the terminal membrane into the bouton and a sequence of events causing the quantal release of neurotransmitters in small multimolecular "packets" from the synaptic vesicles, where the precursors of these transmitters are stored. In brief, a neurotransmitter is synthesized within a neuron, stored and packaged in a vesicle located within a nerve terminal, and released by exocytosis from the vesicle into the synaptic cleft.

Following exocytosis, the vesicle membrane fuses with plasma membrane of the neuron (Fig. 2.2). A new vesicle membrane is formed by pinocytosis (endocytosis) from the plasma membrane and its intermediary structures called cisternae. The coat of the newly formed vesicle is recycled (Fig. 2.2). In addition the neurotransmitters (or their products) and the vesicle membrane are also recycled.

The active *transmitters* include acetylcholine, norepinephrine (noradrenalin), dopamine, and serotonin. The molecules of the neurotransmitters diffuse across the synaptic cleft in less than a millisecond (*synaptic delay*). Depending on the chemical structure of the neurotransmitter and of the receptor chemicals in the receptor sites of the subsynaptic membrane, the resulting permeability changes in the postsynaptic membrane lead to either excitation or inhibition (see below). The response of the postsynaptic membrane (excitation or inhibition) cannot be attributed to the neurotransmitter exclusively; the properties of the receptor are critical. The stimulation of an *excitatory receptor* results in an excitatory response of the subsynaptic membrane, while stimulation of *inhibitory receptors* results in an inhibitory response of the subsynaptic membrane.

Some electrical synapses occur, mainly in invertebrates. In these synapses, the current flow from the axon terminal depolarizes the postsynaptic membrane without need of a chemical transmitter.

Receptor Membrane: Decremental Conduction and Postsynaptic Excitation and Inhibition

The postsynaptic membrane of the dendrite–cell body region in many neurons is known as the *receptor membrane* (*site of synapses*); this membrane propagates its response with decrement rather than in an all-or-none manner. Stimulation of the receptor sites on the cell body and dendrites of a motor neuron evokes a graded response (*generator potential*) which spreads with decrement (not all-or-none) and fades out a short distance before reaching the initial segment of the axon just distal to the axon hillock. The *initial segment* on the axon is the critical site where the action potential is initiated in many axons. The dendrites and cell body are not usually adapted for long-distance transmission but rather for integrating synaptic activity.

Excitation may be explained as a response of the subsynaptic membrane to the neurotransmitter substances that lowers the membrane potential (partial depolarization) to form an *excitatory postsynaptic potential* (*EPSP*). An EPSP is a small, depolarizing potential exhibiting decremental conduction. The excitatory response is associated with Na^+ inrush into the neuron and K^+ outrush from the neuron through the postsynaptic membrane (Fig. 2.5). This graded local change declines slowly and is not conducted.

Whereas excitation is the act of bringing a neuron to a state in which it is more likely to fire, inhibition is the act of preventing a cell from firing. *Inhibition* may be explained as the response of the postsynaptic membrane to a neurotransmitter substance which raises its membrane potential (i.e., hyperpolarization, or increasing the difference in the potential between the cell and the interstitial fluid to, for example, -80 mV). The inhibitory response is associated with Cl^- inrush into the neuron and K^+ outrush from the neuron through the postsynaptic membrane (Fig. 2.5).

The *inhibitory postsynaptic potential* (*IPSP*) opposes an EPSP. A neuron may have many excitatory postsynaptic membrane sites and many inhibitory postsynaptic membrane sites. Both excitatory and inhibitory synapses share the ability to alter the ionic permeability of the postsynaptic membrane.

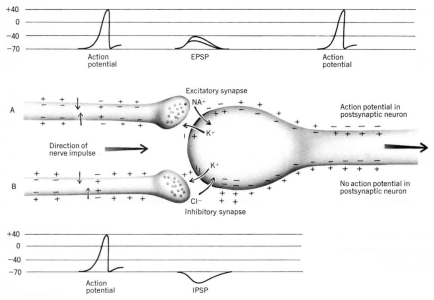

Figure 2.5 Sequences in (A) excitatory and (B) inhibitory transmission from presynaptic neurons (left) across synapses to postsynaptic neuron (right).
(A) The action potential conducted along the presynaptic axon to an excitatory synapse produces an EPSP, which, in turn, can contribute to the generation of an action potential in the postsynaptic neuron.
(B) The action potential conducted along the presynaptic axon to an inhibitory synapse produces an IPSP, which, in turn, suppresses the generation of an action potential in the postsynaptic neuron.

Presynaptic Inhibition

Inhibition may be expressed by a neuron as either postsynaptic (axodendritic or axosomatic synapses) or presynaptic (axoaxonic). *Presynaptic inhibition* operates through an axoaxonic synapse located on an axon proximal to an excitatory (axosomatic or axodendritic) synapse (Fig. 2.3, 2.6). In presynaptic inhibition the presynaptic neuron, acting through an axoaxonic synapse, depolarizes the excitatory (axosomatic or axodendritic) synaptic ending. The excitatory (presynaptic) axon terminal is depolarized by the action of the axoaxonic synapse, so that the action potential, passing down the depolarized ending, cannot, for a few milliseconds, stimulate the release of enough neurotransmitter substance to influence the postsynaptic neuron. In this situation the axoaxonic synapse is actually excitatory, but its effect on the postsynaptic membrane of the axosomatic (or axodendritic) synapse is inhibitory. The inhibitory action results from the depolarization of the presynaptic fibers by axoaxonic synapses and the consequent diminution of transmitter output.

Neuron as an Integrator (Fig. 2.6)

Each neuron is a complex integrator of a mosaic of numerous stimuli streaming into its dendritic field and cell body; the dendrite–cell body complex is specialized to act as a receptor and integrator of stimuli produced by neurotransmitters released by other neurons. Some of the receptive patches (subsynaptic membrane) on the dendrites and cell body are excitatory; others are inhibitory receptive sites. Thus a neuron may be stimulated by excitatory axodendritic and axosomatic synaptic activity and by inhibitory axodendritic and axosomatic synaptic activity. In addition, presynaptic inhibitory activity may indirectly affect some excitatory receptive sites. At any one moment, a neuron may be stimulated by hundreds or even thousands of stimuli on its excitatory and inhibitory subsynaptic membrane patches.

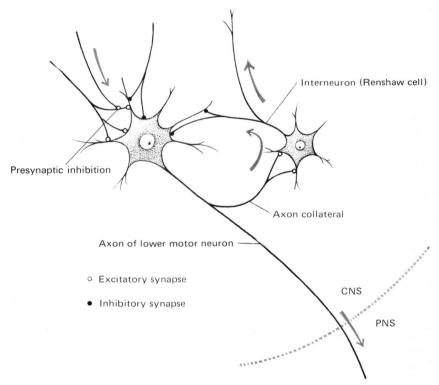

Figure 2.6 The neuron as an integrator (for explanation, see text). The interrupted line represents the boundary between the central nervous system and the peripheral nervous system. Arrows indicate the direction in which nerve impulses are propagated. Neurons from many sources in brain, spinal cord, and body convey influences to each lower motor neuron (Chap. 9), which in turn innervates some voluntary muscle fibers.

Most neurons are under constant *synaptic bombardment.* In this battle-ground of activity, the neuron reacts and may respond. If the summation of the EPSPs exceeds the summation of the IPSPs, the initial segment of the axon may be excited to initiate the production of an action potential in the axon. If the algebraic summation of these potentials (EPSPs and IPSPs) is not sufficient to stimulate the initial segment, an action potential is not generated in the axon. The partial depolarization of the initial segment to the critical voltage is a prerequisite to the generation of an action potential. Thus each dendrite–cell body complex of a neuron is a *miniature integration center,* which will respond with an action potential according to the net effect of the excitatory and inhibitory synaptic activity on the receptive membrane of the neuron. The axon is the vehicle for signaling coded information, via action potentials and synapses, from the dendrite–cell body complex to other neurons or effectors (muscle or gland cells).

Each postsynaptic membrane of the signaled neurons and effectors contains upward of hundreds and thousands of receptors sites, macro-molecular proteins which are specialized decoders. Each receptor site re-sponds to a given stimulus in its own probably predetermined way. For example, acetylcholine is an excitatory agent at a motor end-plate (contrac-tion of voluntary muscle) and an inhibitory agent at the vagus nerve–heart synapses (decrease in heart rate, Chap. 18).

A neuron may in turn be influenced by its own activity through a *negative feedback loop* involving an interneuron (Fig. 2.6). Such an inter-neuron, called a *Renshaw cell,* is intercalated between an axon collateral branch of a lower motor neuron of the spinal cord and the dendrite–cell body region of the same motor neuron and other motor neurons. The axon collateral terminates at an excitatory synapse on the Renshaw cell; the axons of this cell have, in turn, inhibitory synaptic connections with the parent lower motor neuron (Chap. 9).

FIRST-ORDER NEURONS

The sensory or afferent neurons conveying information from the external and internal environment via the peripheral nerves to the CNS have a different structural organization from other neurons (Figs. 5.4 and 17.1). Most of the first-order neurons, called *unipolar* or *pseudounipolar neurons,* are present in all spinal nerves and most cranial nerves. The first-order sensory neurons of the olfactory, optic, and vestibulocochlear systems are *bipolar neurons.* A unipolar neuron has only one process (which, in turn, divides) extending from the cell body, whereas a bipolar neuron has two processes extending from the cell body. No synaptic junctions are associated with the cell bodies of these neurons.

The peripheral telodendritic endings of these fibers—many of which are associated with specialized sensory receptors such as rods and cones in the retina, organ of Corti in the ear, and neuromuscular spindles within muscles—compose the receptive portion of the neurons; this short portion propagates by decremental conduction (generator potential) for a short distance. Except for the short receptive portion, the rest of the process (or processes) propagates action potentials by nondecremental, all-or-none conduction, either as myelinated or unmyelinated fibers, which terminate as axodendritic and axosomatic synaptic junctions within the CNS.

The cell bodies of the first-order neurons are located in the dorsal root ganglia of the spinal nerves (Fig. 17.1) and the sensory ganglia of the cranial nerves (Fig. 12.1). The bipolar cells in the nasal mucosa (olfactory system) and in the retina (visual system) are also first-order neurons.

Chapter 3

Blood Circulation

A copious blood supply is required to sustain the ever-active brain, which gets about one-fifth of the blood pumped by the heart and consumes about 20 percent of the oxygen utilized by the body. Roughly 800 ml of blood flows through the brain each minute, with 75 ml present in the brain at any moment. It takes about 7 s for a drop of blood to flow through the brain from the internal carotid artery to the internal jugular vein. The necessity for this continuous flow is that the brain stores only minute amounts of glucose and oxygen and derives its energy almost exclusively from the aerobic metabolism of glucose delivered by the blood. Each day the brain utilizes about 400 kcal, or about one-fifth of a 2,000-kcal diet. Paradoxically, this blood circulation is minimal; consciousness is lost if the blood supply is cut off for less than 10 s. The demand for blood is the same whether one is resting, sleeping, thinking, or daydreaming.

ARTERIAL SUPPLY

The arterial blood supply to the brain is derived from two pairs of trunk arteries: (1) the vertebral arteries and (2) the internal carotid arteries (Figs. 3.1 and 14.1).

Vertebral Vertebral arteries enter the cranial cavity through the foramen magnum and become located on the anterolateral aspect of the medulla. They unite at the pontomedullary junction to form the *basilar artery*, which continues to the midbrain level, where it bifurcates to form the paired *posterior cerebral arteries*. The branches of the vertebral and basilar arteries supply the medulla, pons, cerebellum, midbrain, and caudal diencephalon, while each posterior cerebral artery supplies part of the caudal diencephalon and the medial aspect (and adjacent lateral aspect) of the occipital lobe including the primary visual cortex (area 17) and the inferior posterior temporal lobe. The branches of the vertebral and basilar arteries that supply the medial aspect of the brainstem adjacent to the midsagittal plane are called *paramedian arteries* (*anterior spinal artery, paramedian branches of the basilar artery*); those that supply the anterolateral aspect of the brainstem are called *short circumferential arteries* (*branches of the vertebral artery, short pontine circumferential branches of the basilar artery*); and those that supply the posterolateral and posterior aspect of the brainstem and cerebellum are the *long circumferential branches* (*posterior spinal artery, posterior inferior* PICA *cerebellar artery, anterior inferior cerebellar artery, superior cerebellar artery,* Fig. 14.1).

Internal Carotid Each internal carotid artery passes through the cavernous sinus as the S-shaped carotid siphon and then divides, level with and lateral to the optic chiasma, into two terminal branches: (1) the *anterior cerebral artery*, which supplies the orbital and medial aspect of the frontal lobe and medial aspect of the parietal lobe, and (2) the *middle cerebral artery*, which passes laterally between the temporal lobe and insula and divides into a number of branches supplying the lateral portions of the orbital gyri and the frontal, parietal, and temporal lobes. The peripheral branches of the middle cerebral arteries anastomose on the lateral surface of the cerebrum with the peripheral branches of the anterior and posterior cerebral arteries. Branches of the middle cerebral artery and the choroidal arteries penetrate into the cerebrum to supply the basal ganglia, most of the diencephalon, internal capsule, and adjacent structures; these central or ganglionic branches (e.g., striate arteries) and the choroidal arteries are variable in their extent and in their anastomotic connections. Other branches of the internal carotid arteries include the *ophthalmic artery* (to the orbit), the *anterior choroidal artery* (to the arc structures adjacent to the choroidal fissure; see Chap. 4), and the *posterior communicating artery* (joins posterior cerebral artery).

Circle of Willis Although the *vertebral-basilar arterial tree* and the *internal carotid arterial tree* are essentially independent, there are some anastomotic connections between the two systems (e.g., between the terminal branches of posterior cerebral arteries and those of the anterior and middle

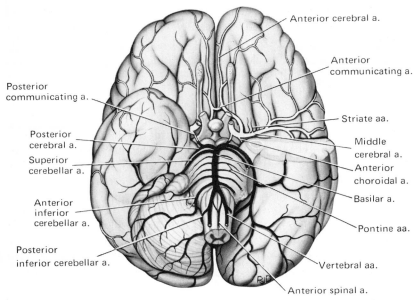

Anterior cerebral a.

Anterior communicating a.

Posterior communicating a.

Striate aa.

Posterior cerebral a.

Middle cerebral a.

Superior cerebellar a.

Anterior choroidal a.

Basilar a.

Anterior inferior cerebellar a.

Pontine aa.

Posterior inferior cerebellar a.

Vertebral aa.

Anterior spinal a.

Figure 3.1 Major arterial supply to the brain. The vertebral–basilar–posterior cerebral arterial tree is indicated as solid black vessels and the paired middle cerebral arterial trees are indicated as white vessels. The circle of Willis includes some arteries of both trees.

cerebral arteries). The *cerebral arterial circle of Willis* is an arterial crown in which the two systems are connected by the small posterior communicating arteries (Fig. 3.1). The circle is completed by the anterior communicating artery which connects the two anterior cerebral arteries. There is actually little exchange of blood through these communicating arteries; the circle of Willis may act as a safety valve when differential pressures are present among these arteries.

The arteries meeting at the cerebral arterial circle of Willis form branches comparable to those of the basilar artery. Thus, (1) the anterior, middle, and posterior cerebral arteries are actually long circumferential arteries; (2) the subbranches (e.g., striate arteries, Fig. 3.1) of these three major cerebral arteries close to the circle of Willis are short circumferential branches; and (3) the small medial arteries from the circle of Willis are paramedian branches.

Anastomotic connections within the vertebral and internal carotid systems are extensive in the brain. Those among the large branches of the superficial arteries on the surface are usually physiologically effective, so that occlusion need not result in any impairment of blood supply to the neural tissues. Rich anastomoses do exist among the capillary beds of adjacent arteries within the substance of the brain, but occlusions of these arteries are often followed by neural damage, because the anastomotic connections may not be sufficient to allow adequate blood to reach the deprived region rapidly enough to meet its high metabolic requirements.

VENOUS DRAINAGE

The veins draining the brainstem and cerebellum roughly follow the arteries to these structures. On the other hand, the veins draining the cerebrum do not usually form patterns which parallel its arterial trees. In general, the venous trees in this region have short, stocky branches which come off at right angles, resembling the silhouette of an oak tree.

Dural Sinuses Venous anastomoses are extensive and effective between the deep veins within the brain and the superficial surface veins (Fig. 3.2). The veins of the brain drain into superficial venous plexuses and the dural sinuses. The *dural (venous) sinuses* are valveless channels located between two layers of the dura mater. Most venous blood ultimately drains into the *internal jugular veins* at the base of the skull.

The blood from the cortex on the upper, lateral, and medial aspects of

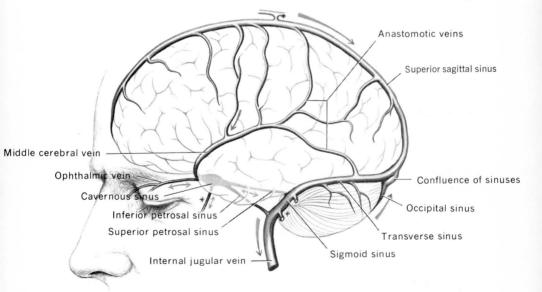

Figure 3.2 Major vessels of the venous drainage of the brain. Arrows indicate direction of blood flow. Depending upon the intracranial pressure, the blood in some vessels can flow in either direction.

the cerebrum drains into the *superior sagittal (dural) sinus* to the occipital region and then to the *right lateral* and *sigmoid sinuses* into the *right internal jugular vein*. All dural sinuses receive blood from veins in the immediate vicinity.

The deep cerebral drainage is to the region of the *foramina of Monro* where the paired internal cerebral veins (located posterior to choroid plexus of third ventricle) extend to the region of the pineal body, where they join to form the *great vein of Galen*. Blood then flows, successively, through the *straight dural sinus* (located on midline within tentorium, which is dura mater located between the cerebellum and the occipital lobe), *left lateral sinus,* and *sigmoid sinus* before draining into the *left internal jugular vein*.

Some blood from the base of the cerebrum drains into the *superior* and *inferior petrosal sinuses* and then flows into either the *sigmoid sinus* or the *cavernous sinus* in the region of the hypothalamus (on the sides of the sphenoid bone). The cavernous sinus is connected via the basilar venous plexus with the venous plexus of the vertebral canal.

Emissary Veins   Some dural sinuses connect with the veins superficial to the skull by *emissary veins*. These veins act as pressure valves when intracranial pressure is raised and are also routes for spread of infection into the brain case (infection in the nose may spread via an emissary vein high in the nose into the meninges and may result in meningitis). The cavernous sinus is connected with emissary veins, including the ophthalmic vein, which extends into the orbit.

Chapter 4

Meninges, Ventricles, and Cerebrospinal Fluid

only this page

MENINGES

The *meninges* are the three layers of connective tissue membranes that surround and protect the soft brain and spinal cord (Fig. 4.1). Each of these layers—pia mater, arachnoid, and dura mater—is a separate, continuous sheet; thin trabeculae extend from the arachnoid to pia mater.

The *pia mater* is intimately attached to the brain and spinal cord, following every sulcus and fissure. It is a vascular layer through which pass blood vessels that nourish the neural tissue.

The *arachnoid* is a thin, avascular, delicate layer, which does not follow each indentation of the brain but rather skips from crest to crest. The *subarachnoid* space between the pia mater and the arachnoid contains cerebrospinal fluid and large blood vessels. Several large spaces called *cisterns* are enlarged in the subarachnoid space. The *cisterna magna (cerebellomedullaris)* is located dorsal to the medulla and inferior to the cerebellum. The *pontine* and *interpeduncular cisterns* are located on the anterior brainstem, and the *superior cistern* is located posterior to the midbrain. The

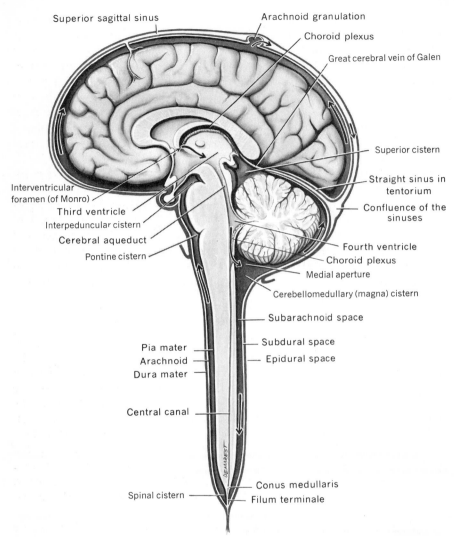

Figure 4.1 Drawing illustrating the meninges, ventricles, subarachnoid spaces, and cisternae. Arrows indicate the normal direction of flow of the cerebrospinal fluid.

lumbar cistern is located caudal to the spinal cord (lumbar-2 to sacral-2 vertebral levels).

The tough, nonstretchable *dura mater* consists of two layers in the head—the outer and inner dura mater. The bony skull and dura mater form an inelastic envelope enclosing the CNS, cerebrospinal fluid, and blood vessels. This inelasticity permits but a slight increase in the cranial contents;

the concept that the volume of the intracranial contents cannot change is the basis of the Monro-Kellie doctrine (see below under "CSF Pressure"). The *outer dura mater* is actually the periosteum of the skull. The *inner dura mater* is a thick membrane which extends (1) between the two cerebral hemispheres in the midsagittal plane as the *falx cerebri* and (2) between the occipital lobe and the cerebellum as the *tentorium.* The *subdural space* is the potential thin space located between the inner dura mater and the arachnoid. The film of fluid in the subdural space is not cerebrospinal fluid.

In head injuries, bleeding may occur into the subarachnoid space (*subarachnoid hemorrhage*), into the subdural space (*subdural hemorrhage*), and between the outer dura mater and the skull (*extradural hemorrhage*). An extradural hemorrhage may result from bleeding meningeal vessels after a fracture of the skull. A subdural hemorrhage may be caused by the tearing of veins crossing the subdural space, which may follow after the sudden movement of cerebral hemispheres relative to the dura and skull. A subarachnoid hemorrhage may result from the rupture of an aneurysm in a branch of the internal carotid or vertebral arteries; the presence of bloodstained cerebrospinal fluid obtained from a lumbar puncture into the lumbar cistern is confirmatory.

VENTRICLES

The *ventricular system* is a series of cavities within the brain, lined by ependyma and filled with cerebrospinal fluid (CSF). The ependyma is a simple cuboidal epithelial layer of glial cells. Each cerebral hemisphere contains a *lateral ventricle,* each of which is continuous through one of the paired foramina of Monro with the *third ventricle* of the diencephalon (Fig. 4.2). The third ventricle is continuous with the tubelike *cerebral aqueduct* (or *iter*) of *Sylvius* of the midbrain, and the latter with the *fourth ventricle* of the pons and medulla. The lateral ventricle is subdivided into four parts: anterior horn in the frontal lobe (rostral to foramen of Monro), body in the parietal lobe, inferior horn in the temporal lobe, and occipital horn in the occipital lobe.

Each ventricle contains a *choroid plexus*—a rich network of blood vessels of the pia mater which are intimately related to the ependymal lining of the ventricles. The membrane formed by the pia mater, its vascular network, and ependyma is called the *tela choroidea.* The choroid plexus of each lateral ventricle is located in the body and inferior horn; it is continuous through a foramen of Monro with the unpaired choroid plexus of the roof of the third ventricle. The choroid plexus of the fourth ventricle is located in the roof of the medulla, in which there are three foramina by which CSF escapes from the fourth ventricle into the cisterna magna. The two lateral openings are the *foramina of Luschka,* and the medial opening is the *foramen of Magendie.*

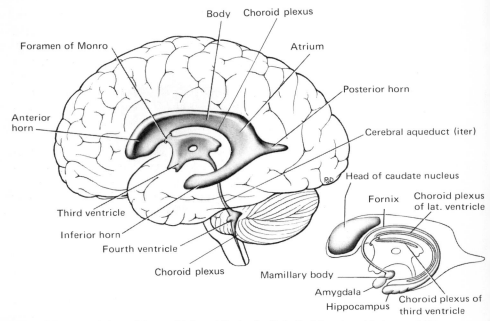

Figure 4.2 Lateral view of the ventricles of the brain. Note that the choroid plexus of the lateral ventricle, the hippocampus-fornix complex, and the caudate nucleus parallel the curvature of the lateral ventricle. The caudate nucleus is cut off just behind its head in this view.

Neural Structures Paralleling the Arc of the Lateral Ventricle

The arc-shaped lateral ventricle follows the curve of the central axis of the frontal, parietal, and temporal lobes. Several important structures trace this arc: (1) caudate nucleus, (2) choroid plexus of the lateral ventricle, (3) hippocampus-fornix system (from the hippocampus in the temporal lobe, fibers of the fornix curve until they terminate in the mamillary bodies of the hypothalamus), and (4) amygdaloid body–stria terminalis system [from the amygdaloid body in the anterior temporal lobe, fibers of the stria terminalis curve until they terminate in the septal area of limbic lobe (Fig. 4.2)].

CEREBROSPINAL FLUID

The *cerebrospinal fluid* is a crystal-clear, colorless solution which looks like water and is found in the ventricular system and the subarachnoid space. The brain and spinal cord actually float in the medium; the 1,400-g brain has a net weight of 50 to 100 g while suspended in the CSF. The brain is "shock-mounted" in the CSF and is thus able to stand the stresses incurred during movements of the head. When fluid is removed, the patient suffers intense pain and excruciating headache with each movement of the head. These painful symptoms persist for a few days until the CSF is naturally replaced.

The volume of CSF in the average adult is estimated to be about 125 ml (25 ml in ventricles and 75 ml in the lumbar sac, or cistern) with 50 to 700 ml said to be formed per day in man. Most of the CSF is formed in the choroid plexuses by active transport and dialysis from the blood; its composition is modified by active transport of elements from adjacent tissues during its passage through the ventricles and subarachnoid spaces. The CSF consists of water; small amounts of protein; gases in solution (oxygen and carbon dioxide); sodium, potassium, and chloride ions; glucose; and a few white blood cells (mostly lymphocytes). Because the CSF is isotonic to blood plasma, it has been characterized as a cell-free, protein-free ultrafiltrate of blood.

Flow of CSF

After its formation at the choroid plexuses and in the ventricular surfaces, there is a bulk flow of CSF through the ventricular system, the subarachnoid spaces, and cisterns surrounding the CNS before entering the blood systemic circulation. The CSF travels from the lateral ventricles through the foramina of Monro into the third ventricle, through the narrow cerebral aqueduct into the fourth ventricle, through the paired apertures of Luschka and the median aperture of Magendie within the tela choroidea in the roof of the fourth ventricle into the cisterna magna, and then slowly circulates rostrally through the subarachnoid space to the region of the superior sagittal venous sinus at the top of the skull. Most of the CSF enters the blood by bulk flow through narrow channels in the arachnoid villi (spongelike structures between subarachnoid space and superior sagittal sinus); a small amount may pass out along nerve roots. The unidirectional flow through the arachnoid villi into the dural sinuses occurs because the villi act as pressure-sensitive valves. When the CSF pressure exceeds the venous pressure, the valves open; when the CSF pressure is reduced below the venous pressure, reflux of blood from the sinus to subarachnoid space is prevented as the valves close.

CSF Pressure

The CSF pressure is lower than blood pressure. In the individual lying on his side, the pressure varies from 60 to 180 mm of water throughout the subarachnoid space. In the seated subject the pressure may rise to between 200 and 300 mm of water in the lumbar cistern, reach zero in the cisterna magna, and go below atmospheric pressure in the ventricles. Fluctuations in the pressure occur in response to phases of the heartbeat and the respiratory cycle. These shifts occur because the rigid box of dura and skull does not yield, so that the intracranial pressure changes if additions or subtractions to the intracranial contents occur (*Monro-Kellie doctrine*).

An obstruction to the normal passage of CSF results in a backup of CSF fluid and an increase in intracranial pressure. Because the CSF extends to the optic disk (optic nerve head, blind spot) of the subarachnoid space within the dural sleeve along the optic nerve, an elevated CSF pressure results in dilated retinal veins and forward thrust of the optic disk beyond the level of the retina. This *papilledema,* or so-called "choked disk," can be observed during an inspection of the fundus of the eye with an ophthalmoscope. A persistent papilledema may result in damaged optic nerve fibers.

X-RAY STUDY OF THE BRAIN

Ventriculography

The ventricles and the subarachnoid space, when they contain air, can be visualized on an x-ray plate. This is accomplished after some CSF is withdrawn and replaced by air, which acts as a contrast medium. The air is introduced by passing a needle either directly into the ventricle or between the lower two lumbar vertebrae (*spinal tap*) into the lumbar cistern (caudal to the spinal cord). The air in the lumbar region can ascend and outline the subarachnoid space of the spinal and cranial cavities (by *pneumoencephalography*); it can also pass through the foramina of Magendie and Luschka to outline the entire ventricular system (in a *ventriculogram*) by serial radiograms (x-rays) taken as the subject is slowly rotated through 360° in a special apparatus.

Angiography

Angiography (arteriography) is the method by which blood vessels—usually arteries—are visualized radiographically following the injection of a nontoxic radiopaque substance into an artery. In cerebral angiography, the sites for the injection of such substances are generally the internal carotid or the vertebral arteries. Injections into the former outline the anterior and middle cerebral arteries, while injections into the latter outline the basilar artery and its major branches, including the posterior cerebral arteries. Angiography is used to outline aneurysms and anomalous arrangements of certain arteries. By changes in the usual arterial patterns, the sites of edema, hemorrhage or tumors may be pinpointed.

Spinal Cord

ANATOMIC ORGANIZATION

The cylindrical spinal cord is located in the upper two-thirds of the vertebral canal of the bony vertebral column. It extends from the foramen magnum at the base of the skull to a cone-shaped termination, the *conus medullaris,* usually located at caudal level of the first lumbar centrum. The nonneural *filum terminale* continues caudally as a filament from the conus medullaris to its attachment in the coccyx (see Fig. 4.1).

The spinal cord is surrounded by three meningeal sheaths which are continuous with those encapsulating the brain. All three meningeal sheaths invest the spinal nerve roots emerging from the spinal cord and are continuous with the connective tissue sheath of the peripheral nerves.

The vascular *pia mater* is intimately attached to the spinal cord, its roots, and the filum terminale. The nonvascular *arachnoid* extends caudally to the sacral-2 vertebral level where it merges with the filum terminale. The *subarachnoid space,* which is filled with CSF and blood vessels, surrounds the spinal cord and is called the *lumbar cistern* between the conus medullaris and the sacral-2 level (Fig. 4.1). The roots of the lumbar and sacral spinal nerves "float" within the CSF of the lumbar cistern. To avoid injury to the spinal cord during removal of CSF, spinal taps into the lumbar cistern are made in the lower lumbar region.

The *dura mater* and the capillary-thin *subdural space* (not containing CSF) surround the arachnoid and merge with the filum terminale. The spinal cord is suspended from the dura mater by a series of 20 to 22 pairs of *denticulate ligaments,* which are flanges extending laterally from the pia mater to the dura mater. The attachment to the dura mater is between two successive spinal nerves. The ligaments are oriented rostrocaudally in a frontal plane between the dorsal and ventral roots.

Between the dura mater (equivalent to inner dura mater surrounding the brain) and the periosteum of the vertebral column (equivalent to outer dura mater surrounding the brain) is the *epidural space* with its venous plexuses and fat. The epidural space caudal to the sacral-2 level is the site for the injection of anesthetics used to modify sensory input (e.g., saddle block for painless childbirth).

Blood Supply

The variably sized spinal arteries are branches of the vertebral, cervical, thoracic, and lumbar arteries. Each artery passes through an intervertebral foramen and divides into an anterior and a posterior spinal root (*radicular arteries*) which form an anastomotic plexus on the surface of the spinal cord. Venous drainage is via a venous plexus, and veins roughly parallel the arterial tree. The large spinovertebral venous plexus is continuous rostrally with that surrounding the brain. An elevation in the venous pressure and the CSF pressure occurs by impeding the outflow of venous blood into the systemic circulation; this results when the pressure in the thoracic and abdominal cavities increases while one is lifting a heavy object or coughing.

SPINAL ROOTS AND PERIPHERAL NERVES

The spinal cord receives its input and projects its output via nerve fibers in the spinal rootlets and roots, spinal nerves, and their branches (Fig. 17.1). Nerve fibers emerge from the spinal cord in a paired, uninterrupted series of dorsal (input, sensory, afferent) and ventral (output, motor, efferent) rootlets which join to form 31 pairs of *dorsal* and *ventral roots.* In the vicinity of an intervertebral foramen, a dorsal root and a ventral root meet to form a *spinal nerve,* which supplies the innervation of a segment of the body. In all, there are 8 pairs of cervical (C); 12 of thoracic (T); 5 of lumbar (L); 5 of sacral (S); and 1 of coccygeal (Co) roots and nerves (Fig. 5.1). (Cervical-1 and coccygeal-1 usually have only ventral roots.)

The thoracic, lumbar, and sacral nerves are numbered after the vertebra

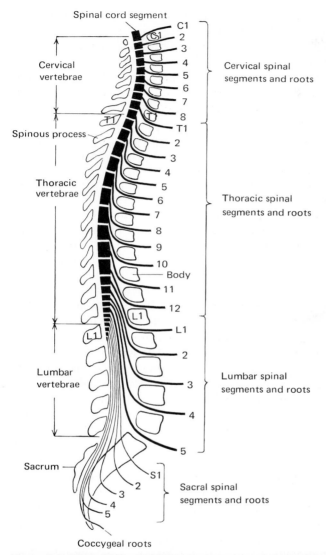

Spinal cord segment

Cervical
vertebrae

Cervical spinal
segments and roots

Spinous process

Thoracic
vertebrae

Thoracic spinal
segments and roots

Body

Lumbar
vertebrae

Lumbar spinal
segments and roots

Sacrum

Sacral spinal
segments and roots

Coccygeal roots

Figure 5.1 Diagram illustrating the topographic relations of the spinal cord segments, spinous processes, and bodies of the vertebrae, intervertebral foramina, and spinal nerves. Refer to Table 5.1. Each spinal cord segment (except upper cervical segments) is located at a higher vertebral level than the site of the emergence of its spinal nerve through the intervertebral foramen. (*Adapted from W. Haymaker, Bing's Local Diagnosis in Neurological Diseases. Mosby, St. Louis, 1969.*)

41

Table 5.1

Spinous process of vertebra	Interspace between vertebral bodies*	Spinal cord segment
C1		C1–2
C6	C6	T1
T10	T10	L1
T12	T12	S1
	T12–L1	All sacral and coccygeal levels
	S2 or S3	Caudal termination of subarachnoid space
	Coccyx	Termination of filum terminale

*Named from centrum of vertebra above interspace.

just rostral to the intervertebral foramen through which they pass (for example, T4 nerve emerges below T4 vertebra); the cervical nerves are numbered after the vertebra just caudal (for example, C7 nerve is rostral to C7 vertebra). Because the spinal cord is much shorter than the bony vertebral column, (1) the spinal nerves emerge from the vertebral column at levels below the spinal cord segments from which their corresponding roots leave the spinal cord (Table 5.1 and Fig. 5.1), and (2) the lumbar and sacral nerves develop long roots which extend as the *cauda equina* (horse's tail) within the lumbar cistern.

The cord is enlarged in those segments that innervate the upper extremities—called the *cervical (brachial) enlargement,* which extends from C5 to T1 spinal levels—and in those segments that innervate the lower extremities—called the *lumbosacral enlargement,* which extends from L3 to S2.

Dorsal Roots

The *dorsal (sensory) roots* consist of the afferent fibers (root fibers) that convey input from the sensory receptors in the body via the spinal nerves to the spinal cord. The cell bodies of these neurons are located in the *dorsal root ganglia* within the intervertebral foramina. The fibers of the dorsal root of each spinal nerve supply the sensory innervation to a skin segment known as a *dermatome* (Fig. 5.2 and Table 5.2). There is usually no C1 or Co1 dermatome. Adjacent dermatomes overlap, so that the loss of one dorsal root results in diminished sensation (not a complete loss) in that dermatome (see Chap. 6).

The afferent fibers are classified, first, by their general distribution into (1) *general somatic afferent (GSA) fibers* conveying influences from sensors in the extremities and body wall, and (2) *general visceral afferent (GVA) fibers* conveying influences from the viscera (e.g., circulatory system); and second, by their conduction velocities into group I fibers with velocities of 70 to 120

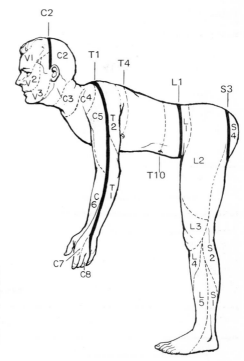

Figure 5.2 Dermatomal (segmental) innervation of the skin. Refer to Table 5.2. The trigeminal nerve is represented by the ophthalmic division (V1), maxillary division (V2), and mandibular division (V3). (*Adapted from W. Haymaker, Bing's Local Diagnosis in Neurological Diseases. Mosby, St. Louis, 1969.*)

meters per second, group II fibers, 30 to 70 meters per second; group III fibers, 12 to 30 meters per second; and group IV fibers, 0.5 to 2 meters per second. Influences from the primary sensory (annulospiral) endings of the neuromuscular spindles are conveyed via group Ia fibers (see below); from Golgi tendon organs via group Ib fibers; from encapsulated skin and joint

Table 5.2

Dorsal spinal root	Body region innervated*
C2	Occiput
C4	Neck and upper shoulder
T1	Upper thorax and inner side of arm
T4	Nipple zone
T10	Umbilical girdle zone
L1	Inguinal region
L4	Great toe, lateral thigh, and medial leg
S3	Medial thigh
S5	Perianal region

*Dermatome and region to which radicular pain is referred.

Table 5.3

Ventral spinal root	Muscles innervated
C5–6	Biceps brachii (flexes elbow)
C6–8	Triceps brachii (extends elbow)
T1–8	Thoracic musculature
T6–12	Abdominal musculature
L2–4	Quadriceps femoris (knee jerk, patellar tendon reflex)
L5–S1–2	Gastrocnemius (ankle jerk, Achilles tendon reflex)

receptors monitoring touch, pressure, temperature, and joint movements (e.g., Meissner's and Pacinian corpuscles) and secondary sensory (flower-spray) endings of neuromuscular spindles via group II fibers; and from nonencapsulated endings monitoring pain, touch, and pressure via group III and group IV fibers.

Ventral Roots

The *ventral* (*motor*) *roots* consist of efferent fibers (root fibers) that convey output from the spinal cord. They are classified as (1) *general somatic efferent* (*GSE*) *fibers,* which innervate voluntary striated muscles (Table 5.3), and (2) *general visceral efferent* (*GVE*) *fibers,* which convey influences to the involuntary smooth muscles and glands (see Chap. 17).

These fibers are axons of (1) the *alpha motor neurons* which convey impulses at 15 to 120 meters per second to motor end-plates of voluntary muscle fibers; (2) the *gamma motor neurons* which convey impulses at 10 to 45 meters per second to motor endings of intrafusal muscle cells of neuromuscular spindles; and (3) the preganglionic autonomic neurons which convey impulses at 0.3 to 1.5 meters per second to synapses with postganglionic neurons. The alpha and gamma motor neurons are known as *lower motor neurons* (*motoneurons*). Each alpha motor neuron and the muscle fibers it innervates constitute a *motor unit;* such units vary from those innervating 3 to 5 muscle fibers (in the finely controlled eye) to those innervating 1,900 muscle fibers (in the soleus muscle of the leg).

Spinal Cord in Cross Section (Fig. 5.3)

The spinal cord is divided into the gray matter (cell bodies, dendrites, axons, and glial cells) and white matter (myelinated and unmyelinated axons and glial cells). The nerve fibers of the gray matter are oriented in the transverse plane, whereas those of the white matter are oriented in the longitudinal plane parallel to the neuraxis. The gray matter has been parceled anatomically, primarily on the basis of the microscopic appearance of the clustering of cell bodies of neurons in stained sections into nuclei or laminae as follows:

Lamina	Corresponding nucleus
I	Posteromarginal nucleus
II	Substantia gelatinosa
III and IV	Proper sensory nucleus (nucleus proprius)
V	Zone anterior to lamina IV
VI	Zone at base of posterior horn
VII	Zona intermedia (includes intermediomedial nucleus, dorsal nucleus of Clarke, and sacral autonomic nuclei)
VIII	Zone in anterior horn (restricted to medial aspect in cervical and lumbosacral enlargements)
IX	Medial nuclear column and lateral nuclear column

The gray matter is also divided into a *posterior horn* (laminae I through VI), an *intermediate zone* (lamina VII), and an *anterior horn* (laminae VIII and IX). The white matter comprises three columns (*funiculi*): posterior, lateral, and anterior.

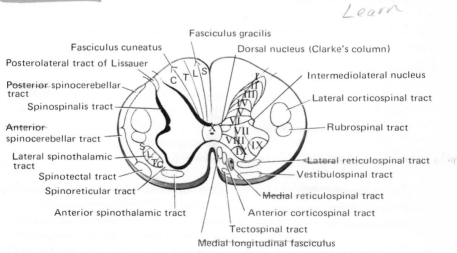

Figure 5.3 Composite diagram of the Rexed laminae (Rexed, 1952) and the tracts of the spinal cord. The ascending tracts are represented on the left and the descending tracts on the right. The lamination of the posterior columns and the lateral spinothalamic tract is indicated. Note somatotopic organization. C, cervical; T, thoracic; L, lumbar; S, sacral.

SPINAL REFLEX ARCS

Reflex arcs are the automatic fixed motor responses to sensory stimuli. These acts are mediated through neuronal linkages called *reflex arcs* (*loops*). Structurally a *spinal somatic reflex arc* comprises sequences that can be summarized in the following manner: (1) A sensory receptor responds to an environmental stimulus. (2) An afferent root neuron conveys influences via the peripheral nerves to nuclei (processing centers, "reflex" centers) within the gray matter of the spinal cord. (3*a*) In the simplest reflex arc the afferent root neuron synapses directly with the lower motor neurons (extensor reflex), or (3*b*) in the more complex reflex arcs the afferent root neuron synapses with interneurons (spinal interneural circuits), which, in turn, synapse with lower motor neurons. (4) A lower (efferent) motor neuron transmits influences to effectors—the striated voluntary muscles. The following examples of reflex arcs are actually "abstractions" of the complex neural circuitry.

Other Myotatic Reflexes

Myotatic reflexes resulting from the stretch of the neuromuscular spindles of any muscle group are known as deep tendon reflexes (DTRs). These include, among others, (1) the biceps reflex—tapping of the biceps brachii tendon results in flexion of the forearm at the elbow, (2) the triceps reflex—tapping of the triceps tendon results in extension of the forearm at the elbow, (3) the quadriceps reflex (knee jerk)—tapping of the quadriceps femoris tendon results in the extension of the leg at the knee, and (4) the triceps sural reflex (ankle jerk)—tapping of the Achilles tendon results in plantar flexion of the foot.

Extensor (Stretch, Myotatic) Reflex (Fig. 5.4)

The simple knee jerk is an *extensor reflex* initiated by the tapping of the relaxed quadriceps femoris muscle. This reflex, essential for the maintenance of muscle tonus, is a *two-neuron* (involving the sequence of an afferent spinal neuron and an efferent spinal neuron), *monosynaptic* (only one set of synapses between the two neurons), *ipsilateral* (reflex arc restricted to one side of the body), and *intrasegmental* (each arc limited to one spinal segment) reflex. The tap stretches the quadriceps muscle and many of its neuromuscular spindles, which are sensitive detectors of muscle length and tension. When stretched, the spindles stimulate group Ia fibers to convey volleys of impulses and, through excitatory synapses, stimulate the ipsilateral alpha (lower) motor neurons which, in turn, results in a quick contraction of the quadriceps muscle. The brisk knee jerk is initiated by the sudden synchronous stretch of many quadriceps neuromuscular spindles. In contrast, the slow contractions maintaining postural muscle tone are initiated by the asynchronous stretching and discharge of many neuromuscular spindles over a period of time.

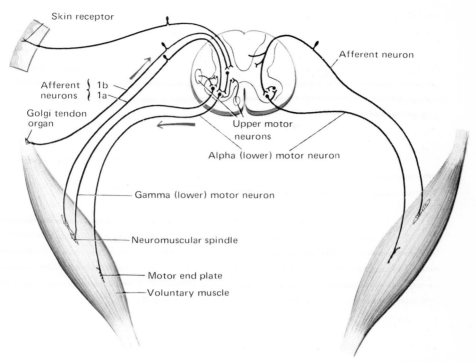

Figure 5.4 The extensor reflex (knee jerk) arc is represented on the right. The gamma reflex loop and the Golgi tendon reflex loop are diagramed on the left. A neuromuscular spindle is an elongated encapsulated sensory receptor composed of 2 to 10 thin, striated muscles (called *intrafusal muscle fibers*), two afferent nerve endings (called *primary* and *secondary sensory endings*), and a gamma motor nerve innervating the intrafusal muscle fibers. Each spindle is oriented with its long axis parallel with the voluntary muscle fibers (called *extrafusal fibers*). The spindle acts as a strain gauge that constantly monitors the tension in the muscle.

Gamma Reflex Loop (Fig. 5.4)

Muscle tone is the residual degree of contraction of voluntary muscles, which exists even when the muscles are "at rest." The extensor reflex acts in the coarse adjustments of muscle tension; fine adjustments and nuances in muscle activity are dependent upon the integrity of the gamma reflex loop. Influences from descending supraspinal pathways from the brain and some peripheral receptors regulate the "set" of the neuromuscular spindles through the gamma motor (fusimotor) neurons. The *gamma loop* comprises, in order: (1) efferent gamma motor neuron, (2) neuromuscular spindle within voluntary muscle, (3) group Ia afferent neuron, (4) alpha motor neuron, and (5) striated muscle fibers. The influences conveyed by the gamma motor neurons can alter the sensitivity of the neuromuscular spindle by altering the length and tension exerted by the intrafusal muscle fibers of the neuromuscular spindles. By increasing the gamma neuron activity, the set of the spindles can be raised to a higher level and can, in turn, increase the firing rate of the Ia fibers stimulating the alpha motor neurons. Many of the descending influences from the brain do not act directly on alpha motor neurons, but rather through the gamma reflex feedback loop through the neuromuscular spindle.

There are two types of gamma motor neurons or systems: *static fusimotor* and *dynamic fusimotor*. The *static* gamma neurons are involved preferentially with tonic reflexes (muscle tone). The rigidity associated with increased tonic stretch reflexes (as in Parkinson's disease, see Chap. 21) may be due to the increased activity of the static fusimotor system. The *dynamic* gamma neurons are involved with the phasic stretch reflexes (e.g., deep tendon reflexes). The spastic signs expressed in upper motor neuron paralysis (Chap. 9) may be primarily due to increased activity of the dynamic fusimotor system. The tonic or static reflexes, characterized by continuous tension and muscular contractions, are involved with the establishment and maintenance of muscle tone for postural purposes. The phasic reflexes are involved in contractions of muscles for movements.

Golgi Tendon Reflex Loop (Fig. 5.4)

This loop comprises (1) the Golgi tendon organ (GTO) in muscle tendons, (2) group Ib afferent fibers, (3) interneurons within the spinal cord, (4) alpha motor neurons, and (5) striated muscle fibers. As the tension within the tendon of a contracting muscle increases, the GTOs increase the number of action potentials conveyed via the Ib afferent neurons to an interneuron pool of the spinal cord. These influences tend to inhibit the activity of the alpha motor neurons. The exquisite balance between the excitatory gamma loop and the inhibitory GTO reflex loop is basic to the precise integration of reflex activity. The GTO reflex loop acts to prevent the overcontraction of the agonist muscle and to facilitate the contraction of the antagonist muscles through reciprocal innervation.

Flexor or Withdrawal Reflex

This flexor reflex is primarily a protective reflex in which the upper extremity, for example, withdraws from a noxious stimulus. Nociceptive stimuli are potent evokers of the superficial or cutaneous reflexes. The reflex circuit of this three-neuron, disynaptic, ipsilateral, intersegmental reflex includes, in order: (1) sensory receptors in the skin, (2) afferent neurons, (3) intersegmental spinal interneurons, (4) alpha motor neurons, and (5) voluntary muscles.

Integration of Spinal Reflexes

Movements are the motor expressions of the integrated activity of many spinal reflex loops and descending supraspinal pathways from the brain (see Chap. 9). The intercalation of spinal interneurons within most reflex loops adds to the complexity and versatility of their activities. *Commissural interneurons* relay influences from one side across the midline to the gray matter of the contralateral side; these are important in crossed reflexes. Intersegmental interneurons project influences from one spinal segment via axons in the fasciculus proprius (spinospinalis tract) to one or more other spinal segments; these neurons are interconnected with commissural interneurons, and together they act as structural substrates in such alternating integrated rhythms of the extremities as walking and running. These interneuronal circuits are crucial to the reciprocal activity of the muscle groups in all movements. For example, in a smooth flexion movement, the flexor muscle group (agonist muscles) contracts while the extensor muscle groups (antagonistic muscles) relax synchronously. Intercalated interneurons within the reflex loops integrate the excitatory (facilitatory) and inhibitory stimuli influencing the lower motor neurons to ensure the precise reciprocal innervation of the agonist and antagonist muscle groups.

Chapter 6

Pain and Temperature

SENSE PERCEPTION

Environmental energies from both inside and outside the body stimulate sensory receptors, which are located throughout the organism. Following the transduction of these energies at the receptors, coded information is transmitted as *nerve impulse patterns* (*action potentials, spikes*) via the afferent fibers of the cranial and spinal nerves to nuclei within the CNS for neural processing.

Some of the input may be integrated into spinal reflex loops or arcs. Other inputs may be relayed via *ascending sensory pathways* consisting of groups of nerve fibers (tracts) linking processing centers (nuclei) and eventually reaching the higher centers in the cerebral cortex. These ascending neural influences to the higher processing centers are integrated into both the conscious (e.g., as pain or touch) and the unconscious activities of the higher centers (e.g., as in motor activities expressed by the cerebellum and hypothalamus).

The processing within the nuclei and cortex involves neural interactions among ascending fibers, small interneurons within the nuclei, and descending fibers from higher centers. In general, the ascending sensory pathways relay information from the body to the cerebral cortex via sequences of three neurons with long axons: (1) first-order neuron, which extends from receptors in the body to the spinal cord or brainstem; (2) second-order neuron, which extends from a nucleus in the spinal cord or brainstem to the thalamus; and (3) third-order neuron, which extends from the thalamus to the cerebral cortex. The axon of a second-order neuron often decussates (crosses over) the midline from one side to the other. Interneurons are located between the first- and second-order neurons and between the second- and third-order neurons (Figs. 6.1 and 7.1).

The spinal nerves transmit relatively unprocessed data from receptors monitoring the general senses—pain, cold, warmth, touch, pressure, movement. The succession of processing sites (nuclei and cortex) in the ascending pathways perform the essential transformations for the conscious appreciation of touch, form, shape, texture, wetness, object identification, sounds, and other sensations.

Receptors   The role of receptors (nerve endings) as "crude sensors" is conceived of in two ways. In the *doctrine of specific nerve energies,* each receptor is presumed to be stimulated by one specific modality—hence pain receptor, touch receptor, cold receptor. The *pattern theory of sensation* postulates that a *group* of nerve endings, if adequately stimulated, responds to a specific modality—hence pain spot, touch spot, cold spot. By differential stimulation of the endings within a "spot," various nuances of the sensation are initiated.

Receptors have been variously classified. The *exteroceptors,* located near the body surface, are generally stimulated by external environmental energies. These are sensed as touch, light pressure, pain, temperature, odor, sound, and light. The *proprioceptors* are located in the deep body wall and extremities. Conscious proprioceptors convey such modalities as position sense and movement, and unconscious proprioceptors (Golgi tendon organs and neuromuscular spindles) transmit information utilized in muscle coordination. The *interoceptors* project information from the viscera sensed as pain, cramps, and fullness, and are utilized in vital reflexes (e.g., carotid sinus reflex). *Mechanoreceptors* respond to mechanical stimuli (touch, hearing). *Chemoreceptors* respond to chemical stimuli (taste, smell).

PAIN AND TEMPERATURE PATHWAYS

The nuclei and nerve fibers that process and convey information resulting in the conscious appreciation of pain and temperature are so closely approximated throughout the nervous system that their pathways are collectively

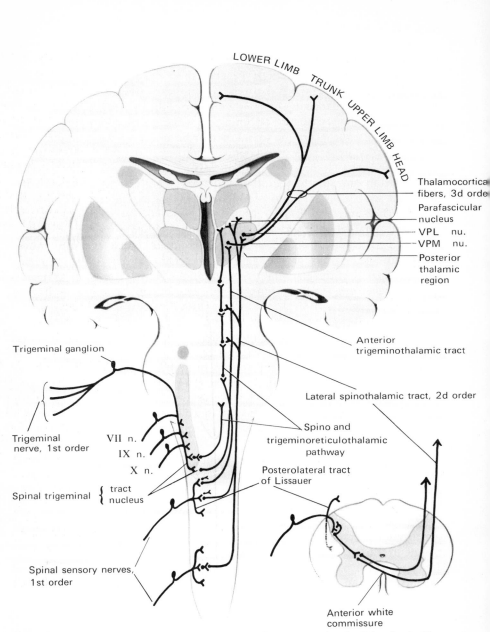

Figure 6.1 The pain and temperature pathways. These comprise the lateral spinotha-lamic tract, spinoreticulothalamic pathway, anterior trigeminothalamic tract, and tri-geminoreticulothalamic pathway. Interneurons are omitted in some nuclei. VPL, ventral posterolateral and VPM, ventral posteromedial of the thalamus; nu, nucleus.

named the pain and temperature pathways (Fig. 6.1). Cutaneous pain sensibility may be tested by pricking the skin with a sharp pin. Thermal sensibility is often evaluated by applying to the body one tube containing ice (40°F), and another containing warm water (110°F). Temperature differences of 5 to 10° are normally detectable.

From the Body and Back of the Head (Occiput) behind the Coronal Plane through the Ears (Fig. 6.1)

Information resulting in the perception of pain is transmitted by free nerve endings and possibly by other receptors in the back of the head (C2 dermatome) and body via first-order thin myelinated and unmyelinated fibers in the peripheral spinal nerves and dorsal spinal roots to the posterior horn of the cord gray matter. "Echo pain"—first and second pain sensations following stimulation (e.g., by a hot object briefly exposed to back of hand)—may be explained by this dual arrangement of high-speed myelinated fibers and low-speed unmyelinated fibers. Temperature is sensed primarily by encapsulated nerve endings and transmitted to the spinal cord via first-order lightly myelinated fibers.

The first-order neurons of pain and temperature with cell bodies located in the dorsal root ganglia enter the spinal cord as the *lateral bundle of the dorsal root,* bifurcate into short ascending and descending branches (one or two spinal segments) within the *posterolateral tract of Lissauer,* branch, and terminate with neurons within the posterior horn (Fig. 6.1). The branches of each fiber terminate in about three adjacent spinal segments. After neural processing within the posterior horn, the long *axons of second-order neurons,* with cell bodies probably in laminae VI and VII, decussate in the *anterior white commissure* (anterior to central canal), ascend as the *lateral spinothalamic tract,* and terminate in the thalamus (*ventral posterolateral nucleus, posterior thalamic region,* and *parafascicular thalamic nucleus;* see Chap. 20).

At successively more rostral spinal levels, new fibers from the higher spinal segments join the lateral spinothalamic tract on its medial aspect; this produces a laminated *somatotopically organized tract* (each body segment has its locale within the tract, Fig. 5.3). As a consequence, pain and temperature fibers from the sacral region are located posterolaterally, and those from the cervical region are located anteromedially. The temperature fibers may be located lateral and posterior to the pain fibers. This lateral spinothalamic tract is also known as the *neospinothalamic tract* (new phylogenetically) or *lateral pain system* (lateral in spinal cord and brainstem). It transmits information perceived as sharp, discriminative, and relatively localized pain sensations. After thalamic processing, the axons of the third-order neuron pass through the posterior limb of the internal capsule and corona radiata before terminating in the second somatic area of the cerebral cortex (some fibers may terminate in the primary somatic area; see Chap. 22).

Pain may be conveyed via the *spinoreticulothalamic pathway system* (Fig. 6.1). Pain fibers of the spinoreticular and lateral spinothalamic tract terminate and synapse within the brainstem reticular formation and are integrated in this diffuse, multisynaptic, multineuronal pathway which terminates in thalamic intralaminar nuclei (parafascicular nucleus and others). This *medial pain system*—also called the *paleospinothalamic system* (phylogenetically old)—is involved with the more diffuse, poorly localized pain sensations.

The lateral spinothalamic tract, anterior spinothalamic tract (see Chap. 7), and the spinoreticulothalamic pathways are often grouped together as the *anterolateral pathways.*

From the Anterior Head (Face, Forehead, Eyeball, and Structures Associated with Orbital, Nasal, Paranasal, and Oral Cavities)

From receptors in the anterior head (anterior to coronal plane through the ears), pain and temperature fibers convey impulses via the three divisions of the trigeminal nerve (ophthalmic, maxillary, and mandibular) and cranial nerves VII, IX, and X (Fig. 6.1). The cell bodies of these first-order fibers are located in the *trigeminal ganglion* (V), the *geniculate ganglion* (VII), and the *superior ganglia* (IX and X). These fibers enter the brainstem and descend as the *spinal trigeminal tract* on the lateral aspect of the lower pons, medulla, and upper two cervical spinal segments. The spinal trigeminal tract is somatotopically organized: the sequence from anterior to posterior includes the fibers from the ophthalmic nerve (most anterior), maxillary nerve, mandibular nerve, and nerves VII, IX, and X (dorsal); fibers from each of these nerves extend to the C2 level. These fibers terminate in the spinal trigeminal nucleus which is located medial to the tract. The spinal trigeminal tract and nucleus are the brainstem's counterpart of the posterolateral tract of Lissauer and substantia gelatinosa of the spinal cord, respectively.

From second-order neurons in the spinal trigeminal nucleus, axons decussate through the lower brainstem reticular formation, ascend near the medial lemniscus as the *anterior trigeminal tract* (*anterior trigeminothalamic tract*), and terminate in the *ventral posteromedial nucleus* of the thalamus and *posterior thalamic region.* Axons of the third-order neurons pass from the thalamus through the posterior limb of the internal capsule and corona radiata before terminating in the head region in the *lower postcentral gyrus* (*primary* and *secondary somatic area;* see Chap. 22). This pathway is included in the *lateral pain system.* Diffuse, poorly localized pain from the head is probably conveyed via the *trigeminoreticulothalamic pathway* of the brainstem reticular formation—*medial pain system*—to thalamic intralaminar (e.g., parafascicular nucleus) nuclei.

PERCEPTION OF PAIN

Pain is primarily a warning signal to the organism; it is often accompanied by withdrawal from a noxious stimulus via the protective flexor reflex. The awareness of pain may be a functional expression of the thalamus. The various nuances of pain (sharp pain, dull pain, headaches) may require the functional activity of the secondary somatic area of the cerebral cortex (see Chap. 22). Descending influences from the cerebral cortex and other centers may modify the perception of pain. The descending fibers terminate in the spinal trigeminal nucleus and posterior horn of the spinal cord; they probably act to modify the input from the periphery.

Pain can be initiated in several ways—by mechanical, thermal, electrical, and chemical stimuli. Three types of pain exist (1) fast-conducted, sharp, prickling pain, (2) slowly conducted, burning pain, and (3) deep, aching pain (in joints, tendons, and viscera).

Referred Pain

Pain of visceral origin is usually vaguely localized. The site of the visceral irritation and the locale where the pain is felt are not necessarily the same. The pain is referred from the visceral source to a corresponding dermatome segment on the body wall or extremity; for example, stimuli from the heart may be referred to the left thoracic wall and inner left upper arm, or stimuli from the jejunum may be referred to the region of the umbilicus. Headaches may be referred from irritation of the meninges, extracranial or intracranial blood vessels, and other sites.

Pain in Dermatomes

A *dermatome* is the sensory segment of the skin innervated by the fibers of one dorsal root. Dermatomes of successive spinal segments overlap. Hence the interruption of one complete dorsal root may result in only the diminution (not loss) of sensation in part of a dermatome. However, the irritation of a dorsal root can produce pain over an entire dermatome (see Fig. 5.2). In herpes zoster (shingles) there is an intense and persistent pain in one or more dermatomes. This pain is a consequence of the activation of pain fibers by varicella zoster virus, which primarily affects one or more dorsal root ganglia. Mechanical compression, e.g., following a slipped disk, of a dorsal root can irritate a dorsal root and produce pain over a dermatome.

Tractotomy

To abolish intractable pain, neurosurgeons may transect the pain tracts in a procedure known as *tractotomy*. After the transection of an anterior quadrant of the spinal cord at some level, the lateral spinothalamic tract and other tracts are interrupted. Pain and temperature on the opposite side of the body beginning one or two levels below the transection should be lost. Bilateral tractotomy of the pain tracts should abolish visceral and somatic intractable pain below the level of the chordotomy. Tractotomy of the descending uncrossed fibers of the spinal trigeminal tract above the level of the obex (medulla) should result in loss of pain and temperature on the same side of the face and nasal and oral cavities (see Chap. 14, "Region of the Cerebellopontine Angle").

Phantom Limb Sensation

The phantom limb is an expression of activity in nuclei deprived of the normal stimulation. An amputee may feel a diffuse pain in his amputated extremity. The phantom limb "moves" easily, even through objects and the remaining or absent limb. The wristwatch, formerly worn, may still be felt on the nonexistent wrist. An explanation is that the nuclear complexes that previously received input from the phantom limb are still present in the nervous system; when these complexes are stimulated in some way, they set in motion neural activities which produce sensations felt as though coming from the absent limb.

Somatotopic Organization of Lateral Spinothalamic Tract

The laminated, somatotopic organization of the lateral spinothalamic tract, with fibers from successively higher levels located anteromedial to those from lower levels, has significance in analyzing distributions of pain sensation (Fig. 5.3). Pressure on the lateral aspect of the cervical spinal cord (e.g., from extramedullary tumor) would interrupt pain and temperature fibers from the contralateral sacral region first and then, as the tumor enlarges, those from lumbar, thoracic, and cervical regions. Pressure from the middle of the spinal cord (central canal region) in the cervical region (e.g., with intramedullary tumor) would interrupt pain and temperature fibers from the contralateral cervical region first and then, as the tumor enlarges, those from the thoracic, lumbar, and sacral regions.

learn whole chapter

Chapter 7

Discriminative General Senses

The *discriminative general senses* include discriminative touch; pressure touch; two-point discrimination; stereognosis; awareness of shape, size, and texture; awareness of movement; position sense; vibratory sense (tuning fork); and weight perception. These modalities are monitored by both exteroceptors and proprioceptors. The receptors are located in the skin, joints, periosteum, tendons, and muscles.

Light touch or tactile sensibility is the sensation felt during the gentle stroking of hairless skin with cotton (Merkel's disk and Meissner's corpuscle are receptors) and movement of hair (peritrichial nerve plexus around hair roots is receptor). The sense of light touch grades gradually into sense of pressure touch.

TACTILE SENSIBILITY (LIGHT TOUCH) PATHWAYS
From the Body and Back of Head (Occiput)

Light touch from the body and the back of the head is conveyed from peripheral receptors via first-order neurons with cell bodies in the dorsal root ganglia of the peripheral nerves to the posterolateral tract of Lissauer, where the fibers bifurcate and ascend and descend several spinal levels before terminating with interneurons of the posterior horn (Fig. 7.1). Some first-order neurons may pass through the medial bundle and terminate in the posterior horn (bypassing the posterolateral tract of Lissauer). Processing occurs within the interneuronal circuits of the posterior horn. The axons of neurons of the second order, with cell bodies presumably in laminae VI and VII, decussate through the anterior white commissure and then ascend as the *anterior spinothalamic tract* and terminate in the *ventral posterolateral nucleus* of the thalamus. This pathway is somatotopically organized, with fibers from the sacral levels located laterally, and those from cervical levels most medially within the tract (Fig. 5.3). In the lower brainstem this tract is located close to the lateral spinothalamic tract. The axons of the neurons of the third order pass through the posterior limb of the internal capsule and the corona radiata before terminating in the postcentral gyrus. After neural processing in this gyrus, pyramidal neurons of cortex project information to the parietal association cortex (see Chap. 22). Light touch is also conveyed via the *posterior column–medial lemniscus pathway* and the *spinocervical thalamic pathway* (see Chap. 8).

From the Anterior Head

Light touch from the head anterior to the coronal plane through the ears is conveyed via neurons of the trigeminal nerve, which enter through the lateral midpons. Some fibers of these neurons terminate in the principal sensory trigeminal nucleus of the pons. Other fibers bifurcate into collaterals which terminate in the principal sensory trigeminal nucleus and other collaterals which descend for a short distance in the spinal trigeminal tract before terminating in the spinal trigeminal nucleus. From cell bodies of neurons of the second order, located in the principal sensory trigeminal nucleus and rostral portion of the spinal trigeminal nucleus, axons *decussate* in the pontine tegmentum and ascend as the *anterior trigeminal tract* (anterior trigeminothalamic tract) before terminating in the *ventral posteromedial thalamic nucleus* (Fig. 7.1). Some axons of second-order neurons of the principal (sensory) trigeminal nucleus ascend as *uncrossed* fibers as the *posterior trigeminal tract* (posterior trigeminothalamic tract) to the ventral posteromedial thalamic nucleus. Axons of the neurons of the third order of this thalamic nucleus then pass through the posterior limb of the internal capsule and corona radiata before terminating in the head region of the postcentral gyrus, whence association fibers project to the association cortex of the parietal lobe (see Chap. 22).

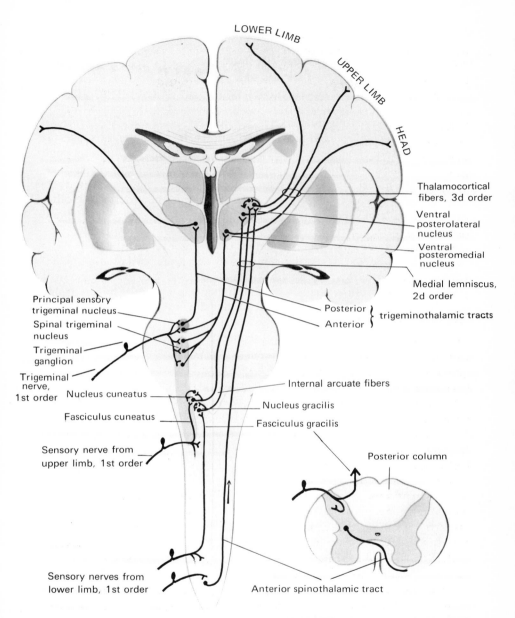

Figure 7.1 The discriminative general sensory pathways. These comprise the anterior spinothalamic tract, posterior column–medial lemniscus pathway, and anterior and posterior trigeminothalamic tracts. Interneurons are omitted in some nuclei.

DISCRIMINATIVE GENERAL SENSES PATHWAYS

From the Body and Back of Head (Occiput)

vibration, position sense

Information perceived as discriminative general senses is conveyed from the peripheral receptors via the fibers of the first-order neurons of the peripheral nerves. Their heavily myelinated fibers enter the spinal cord as the *medial bundle of the dorsal roots* (Fig. 7.1) and branch into collaterals which (1) terminate mainly in laminae III and IV of the posterior horn and (2) ascend in the *posterior white columns (fasciculi gracilis and cuneatus)* before terminating in the nuclei gracilis and cuneatus in the lower medulla. The fibers terminating in the posterior horn are incorporated in the anterior spinothalamic pathway, and those terminating in the ipsilateral nuclei gracilis and cuneatus in the posterior column–medial lemniscal pathway (Fig. 7.1). Collaterals of these fibers are integrated into spinal reflexes.

The fibers of the first-order neurons of the posterior column–medial lemniscal pathway are somatotopically organized (Fig. 5.3). Fibers are added to the posterior column (fasciculi gracilis and cuneatus) on the lateral aspect at each succeeding higher spinal level so that the lamination from posteromedial to lateral in the cervical levels consists, in order, of fibers from the sacral, lumbar, thoracic, and cervical segments of the body. The fibers from the sacral, lumbar, and lower six thoracic levels compose the *fasciculus gracilis,* and those from the upper six thoracic and all cervical levels (includes back of head) compose the *fasciculus cuneatus.* The fibers terminating in the nucleus gracilis originate from below T6, including the lower extremities, and those in the nucleus cuneatus originate from above T6, including the upper extremities. The longest neurons in the body are those of the fasciculus gracilis; they extend without interruption from receptors in the foot through the spinal nerves, dorsal roots (location of their cell bodies), and fasciculus gracilis to the nucleus gracilis.

Neural processing within the nuclei gracilis and cuneatus occurs through the synaptic interactions among the nerve terminals of ascending fibers, intrinsic interneurons, descending corticonuclear fibers from the cerebral cortex (see Chap. 9), and neurons of the second order. The processed information is relayed via the axons of second-order neurons which emerge from the nuclei gracilis and cuneatus, arc anteriorly as the *internal arcuate fibers,* decussate in the lower medulla, ascend as the somatotopically organized *medial lemniscus* (Figs. 11.4 and 11.5), and terminate in the *ventral posterolateral thalamic nucleus.* As it ascends, the medial lemniscus gradually shifts from a medial location in the medulla to a posterolateral location in the upper midbrain. Axons of neurons of the third order of the ventral posterolateral thalamic nucleus pass through the posterior limb of the internal capsule and corona radiata before terminating in the postcentral gyrus, whence association fibers project to the association cortex of the parietal cortex (see Chaps. 20 and 22).

From the Anterior Head

The discriminative general senses from the head anterior to the coronal plane through the ears are conveyed via neurons of the trigeminal nerve which terminate mainly in the principal sensory trigeminal nucleus (Fig. 7.1). The ascending pathways associated with these modalities are similar to those described with tactile sensibility (see "From the Anterior Head" above). The principal sensory trigeminal nucleus is the cranial equivalent for the nuclei gracilis and cuneatus. In these nuclei are located the cell bodies of second-order neurons of the discriminative general senses.

FUNCTIONAL CORRELATIVES

The general sensory pathways conveying pain and temperature, tactile sensibility, and discriminative senses have, with a few exceptions, similar features. The neurons of the first order extend from receptors in the periphery and terminate within nuclei (or laminae) in the ipsilateral half of the spinal cord or brainstem. The cell bodies of these neurons are located in ganglia (with no synapses within them) just outside the CNS: dorsal root ganglia, trigeminal ganglion, geniculate ganglion, and superior ganglia of cranial nerves IX and X. The neurons of the second order have cell bodies in a nucleus on the ipsilateral side and axons that decussate to the contralateral side and ascend as tracts which terminate in the thalamus (ventral posterior nucleus and posterior thalamic region). The neurons of the third order project from the thalamus to the postcentral gyrus (primary somatic area) and adjacent secondary somatic area (Fig. 22.4). Note that the spinothalamic fibers (neurons of the second order) decussate at all levels of the spinal cord, with each fiber crossing at a spinal level near the location of its cell body, whereas all second-order neurons of the posterior column–medial lemniscal pathway have axons that decussate at a common level as the internal arcuate fibers in the lower medulla.

   Light touch may be conveyed via two pathways: (1) the anterior spinothalamic tract (and its cranial equivalent, the anterior trigeminal tract) and (2) the posterior column–medial lemniscal pathway (and its cranial equivalent, the anterior and posterior trigeminal tracts).

   The loss of tactile sensibility is known as *tactile anesthesia.* A diminution in tactile appreciation is called *tactile hypesthesia,* while an exaggeration of the perception of touch, which is often unpleasant, is usually referred to as *tactile hyperesthesia.* The last-mentioned may be accompanied by *paresthesias*—the sensations of numbness, tingling, prickling, and feeling of discomfiture.

Impairment of the Posterior Column–Medial Lemniscal Pathway

The interruption of this discriminative general pathway results in disturbances in the appreciation of certain sensations and in the regulation and control of movements.

The alterations in the appreciation of the discriminative general senses include:

1 Diminution, not loss, of *light touch*. This modality is partially retained because the anterior spinothalamic tract is intact and functional.

2 Loss of *vibratory sense*. The perception of the "buzz" of vibrations is tested by placing the base of a vibrating tuning fork on a joint or bone (e.g., knee, elbow, finger, spinous process of vertebra).

3 *Astereognosis*—loss of the ability to recognize and identify common objects by feel, touch, and handling, but full ability to recognize the same objects by sight. A patient with astereognosis is unable to identify a key, coin, knife, or pencil by touch.

4 Loss of *two-point discrimination*—the ability to recognize two blunt points as two points when applied simultaneously.

5 Loss of *position sense*—the ability to know where a part of the body is located or to appreciate movement of a joint.

The impairment of sufficient proprioceptive input results in unsteady, awkward, and poorly coordinated movements. This "sensory" *ataxia* may be a consequence of lesions in the posterior column–medial lemniscal pathway including the dorsal roots, posterior column (posterior column ataxia), nuclei gracilis and cuneatus, and medial lemniscus. Patients show an unsteady gait while walking or turning; to reduce the unsteadiness, they walk with a broad base. In severe cases the patient may stagger and fall while the eyes are closed. The signs of the ataxia are more pronounced in patients in the dark or with eyes closed. The severity of the symptoms is reduced when the subject can use visual cues; this is consistent with the concept that two of three of the following sources of sensory input are essential for adequate regulation of posture and movement: proprioceptive general senses, vision, and vestibular sense. *Romberg's sign* is often used to detect posterior column ataxia: In the erect position with feet close together, the ataxic patient will sway when the eyes are closed; swaying is reduced or abolished when the eyes are opened.

Chapter 8

Other General Sensory Ascending Tracts

SPINOCEREBELLAR PATHWAYS

The cerebellum requires a continuous flow of information concerning the ongoing dynamics of the muscles, tendons, and joints. This cerebellar input, also called *unconscious proprioception,* is relayed from the body via several pathways, including the posterior and anterior spinocerebellar tracts, cuneo-cerebellar tract, rostral spinocerebellar tract, and spinoreticulocerebellar tract. The peripheral receptors monitoring this information include the neuromuscular spindles, Golgi tendon organs, touch endings, and pressure receptors.

Posterior Spinocerebellar Tract (Fig. 8.1)

The neurons of the first order with cell bodies in dorsal root ganglia convey coded information from stretch receptors directly to the neurons of the second order in the *dorsal nucleus* (*Clarke's column*) of lamina VII. The first-order neurons include groups Ia and II fibers from the neuromuscular spindle and group Ib fibers from the Golgi tendon organs, touch receptors,

63

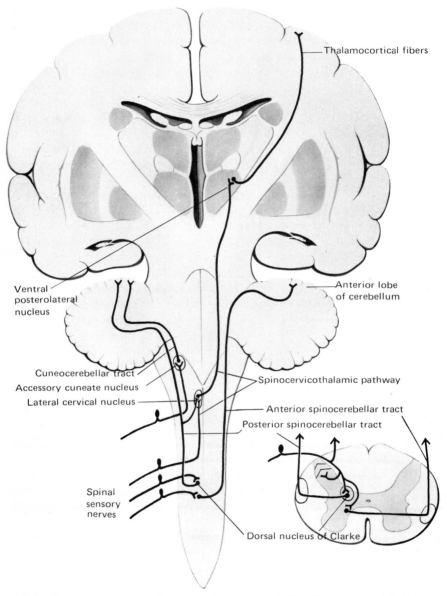

Figure 8.1 Ascending tracts from the spinal cord including the anterior and posterior spinocerebellar tracts, cuneocerebellar tract, and spinocervicothalamic pathway.

and pressure receptors. This monosynaptic pathway then relays from the dorsal nucleus of Clarke (located at levels T1 through L2), via mainly uncrossed fibers, to ascend successively through the posterior spinocerebellar tract and inferior cerebellar peduncle (restiform body, Fig. 11.1) and terminate in the area for the lower extremities in the anterior and posterior lobes of the cerebellum. In brief, the somatotopically organized posterior spinocerebellar tract relays unconscious proprioceptive information from the caudal half of the body and lower extremities to the cerebellar cortex via a two-neuron linkage with synaptic connections in the dorsal nucleus of Clarke. This pathway has a role in the fine coordination of individual muscles during posture and movement.

Anterior Spinocerebellar Tract (Fig. 8.1)

Fibers of neurons of the first order from the flexor reflex receptors and Golgi tendon organs located in the lower half of the body and lower extremities enter the spinal cord via the dorsal roots and terminate monosynaptically with second-order neurons within laminae V, VI, and VII in the thoracic and lumbar levels. Axons of these second-order neurons mainly decussate through the anterior white commissure and ascend as the somatotopically organized *anterior spinocerebellar tract* through the spinal cord, medulla, and superior cerebellar peduncle (Fig. 11.1), before terminating in the lower extremity area of the cerebellar cortex (anterior lobe). This pathway has a role in the general aspects of posture and movements of the entire lower limb.

Cuneocerebellar Tract (Fig. 8.1)

Group Ia and cutaneous afferent fibers of first-order neurons innervating the rostral half of the body and upper extremities pass through the dorsal roots, ascend in the ipsilateral fasciculus cuneatus, and terminate in the *accessory cuneate nucleus* (Figs. 8.1 and 11.4), located lateral to the cuneate nucleus in the lower medulla. Axons from neurons of the accessory cuneate nucleus pass via the *cuneocerebellar tract* through the inferior cerebellar peduncle and terminate in the upper extremity area of the anterior and posterior lobes of the cerebellum. This pathway is the rostral equivalent of the posterior spinocerebellar tract.

Rostral Spinocerebellar Tract

This pathway serves the same role for the rostral half of the body and upper extremities as the anterior spinocerebellar tract for the lower extremities. Although its presence has been established only in cats at present, it is presumed to be present in man. This rostral spinocerebellar pathway relays influences primarily via uncrossed fibers which pass through both the superior and inferior cerebellar peduncles and terminate in the upper extremity region of the cerebellar cortex.

General Aspects of Spinocerebellar Tracts

The anterior and posterior spinocerebellar tracts convey unconscious proprioceptive influences from the caudal half of the body and lower extremities to the cerebellum. The cuneocerebellar and rostrocerebellar tracts convey similar influences from the rostral half of the body and upper extremities to the cerebellum. The posterior spinocerebellar and cuneocerebellar tracts convey information primarily from neuromuscular spindles, Golgi tendon organs, and touch and pressure receptors of the skin, whereas the anterior spinocerebellar and rostral spinocerebellar tracts convey input from large receptive fields of Golgi tendon organs and flexor reflex afferents.

SPINORETICULAR FIBER ROUTES

From cell bodies located in the spinal gray matter of all spinal levels, axons pass into the anterolateral funiculus and ascend mainly as ipsilateral spinoreticular fibers, which terminate in several nuclei of the lower brainstem reticular formation. Some of the ascending influences are integrated into the pain pathways—the spinoreticulothalamic pathway (Fig. 6.1) and the ascending reticular activating system (see Chap. 19). Other ascending fibers terminate in the lateral reticular nucleus (located in the lateral medulla) and other lower brainstem reticular nuclei, which relay influences via the inferior cerebellar peduncle to the cerebellum.

SPINOTECTAL TRACT

The fibers of this tract convey influences from the contralateral spinal gray matter via crossed fibers which ascend adjacent to the lateral spinothalamic tract before terminating in the superior colliculus and nearby midbrain reticular formation. The pathway has been associated with the appreciation of diffuse, poorly localized pain and associated nociceptive feelings related to the "medial" pain system (see Fig. 6.1).

SPINOCERVICOTHALAMIC PATHWAY (SPINOCERVICOLEMNISCAL PATHWAY)

This pathway has an, as yet, unknown role in the transmission of tactile and kinesthetic information to the ventral posterolateral thalamic nucleus and the cerebral cortex (Fig. 8.1). It differs from the spinothalamic and posterior column–medial lemniscal pathways in that an additional relay nucleus—the *lateral cervical nucleus* located in the lower medulla and upper two cervical levels—is interposed between the first-order neurons from the periphery and the neurons projecting to the thalamus. This pathway has been demonstrated in the rhesus monkey and is thus assumed to be a functioning pathway in man. The influences from the afferent fibers of first-order neurons reach the lateral cervical nucleus indirectly via two routes: (1) collateral branches of the posterior spinocerebellar fibers and (2) axons of neurons located in the gray matter of the lumbosacral region (Fig. 8.1). Axons of neurons of the lateral cervical nucleus decussate in the lower medulla, ascend in the brainstem, and terminate in the ventral posterolateral thalamic nucleus.

OTHER ASCENDING FIBERS FROM THE SPINAL CORD

Several ascending systems, each consisting of relatively few fibers, project from the spinal cord to the brain. Among these groupings of fibers, described in man and experimental mammals, are the *spinocortical fibers* terminating in the cerebral cortex, *spinopontine fibers* terminating in the pontine nuclei of the cortico-pontine-cerebellar system (see Chap. 15), and the *spinovestibular fibers* terminating in the lateral vestibular nucleus (see Chap. 13). *Spino-olivary fibers* are probably not present in man and apes. The functional role of these fiber systems is unknown; they may convey influences of significance in certain reflex activities and feedback systems.

Chapter 9

Lower Motor Neurons, Upper Motor Neurons, and Motor Pathways

LOWER MOTOR NEURONS

The voluntary (striated, skeletal) muscles are innervated by *alpha motor neurons,* which have heavily myelinated, fast-conducting axons terminating in the motor end-plates of extrafusal voluntary muscle fibers. Because these are the only neurons innervating these muscles, they function as the *final common pathway,* the final linkage between the CNS and voluntary muscles. The intrafusal voluntary muscles of the neuromuscular spindles are innervated by *gamma motor neurons,* which have lightly myelinated, slow-conducting axons. The alpha and gamma motor neurons are called *lower motor neurons (spinomuscular neurons).* From cell bodies located in nuclei within the CNS (brainstem and spinal cord), the axons of these neurons pass through the cranial and peripheral nerves before terminating at the muscle cells (see Figs. 5.4 and 9.1).

The *lower motor neurons* are the general somatic efferent (GSE) components of the spinal nerves and of cranial nerves III, IV, VI, and XII, and

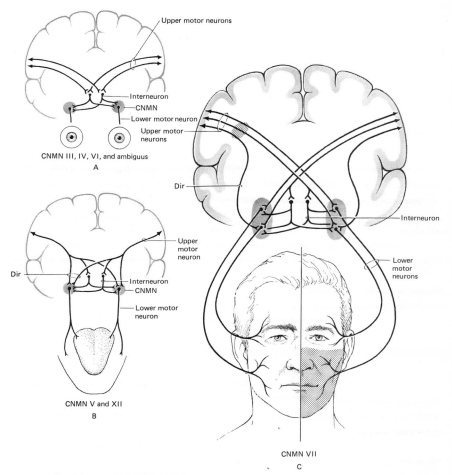

Figure 9.1 The three groups of cranial nerve motor nuclei (CNMN) according to their upper motor neuron (UMN) innervation. (A), *CNMN III, IV, VI, and Ambiguus*. The UMNs exert influences through direct bilateral projections to interneurons, which, in turn, innervate the lower motor neurons (LMN) of these motor nuclei. (B), *CNMN V and XII*. The UMNs exert influences both through (1) indirect bilateral projections to interneurons and (2) direct (Dir) bilateral projections to the LMNs of these motor nuclei. (C), *CNMN VII*. The UMNs exert influences through indirect bilateral projections to LMNs. *Of importance*, (1) the LMNs innervating muscles of upper face and forehead receive direct (Dir) bilateral UMN projections and (2) the LMNs innervating muscles of lower face receive predominantly direct crossed UMN projections. The UMN lesion (shaded) results in a paralysis limited to muscles of contralateral lower face (shaded).

the special visceral efferent (SVE) components of cranial (branchiomeric) nerves V, VII, IX, X, and XI (Chap. 12). The lower motor neurons of the spinal cord are often called *anterior horn motor neurons* (cell bodies located in the anterior horn of the spinal cord) or *motoneurons*. It is important to recognize that lower motor neurons are located in both cranial and spinal nerves.

UPPER MOTOR NEURONS

The facilitatory (excitatory) and inhibitory influences stimulating the lower motor neurons are conveyed via fibers from two general sources: (1) the head and body via the cranial and spinal nerves—information from these sources is integrated in reflex activity, and (2) the brain via descending supraspinal pathways—these are generally called "voluntary" pathways.

The *descending supraspinal pathways* project influences that modify the activity of the lower motor neurons; they are called *upper motor neurons.* These include the neurons and their fibers of (1) the *corticospinal* (*pyramidal*) and *corticobulbar tracts* originating in the cerebral cortex (Fig. 9.1), (2) the *rubrospinal, tectospinal,* and *interstitiospinal tracts* originating in the midbrain, and (3) the *reticulospinal* and *vestibulospinal tracts* originating in the lower brainstem (pons and medulla, Fig. 9.2). Many clinicians refer to the corticospinal tract as the *upper motor neuron tract.*

In contrast to a lower motor neuron, which is present in both the central and peripheral nervous systems, an upper motor neuron is located wholly within the central nervous system. The upper motor neurons have significant roles in the maintenance of posture and equilibrium, control of muscle tone, and reflex activity. In general, the influences conveyed via the descending supraspinal pathways exert their effects (1) on groups of muscles and movements (e.g., flexion, extension, adduction) and not primarily on one specific muscle and (2) reciprocally upon agonist and antagonist muscle groups (e.g., they facilitate flexion and inhibit extension, or inhibit flexion and facilitate extension).

Other Supraspinal Neurons Two other types of descending supraspinal pathways are functionally significant: (1) Some fibers, simply called *corticonuclear fibers,* descend and terminate in the sensory relay nuclei of the ascending pathways (e.g., posterior horn, nuclei gracilis and cuneatus, and spinal trigeminal nucleus). These pathways modulate sensory input and modify the processing within these nuclei. (2) The descending fibers of the autonomic nervous system influence and regulate visceral activity through connections with the preganglionic neurons of the sympathetic and para-

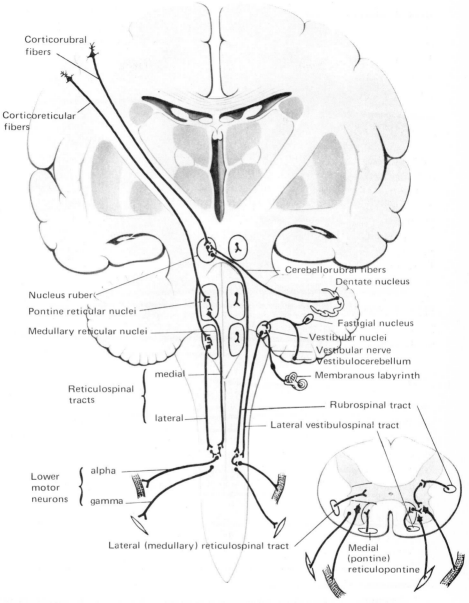

Figure 9.2 Descending motor pathways to the spinal cord including the reticulospinal tracts (corticoreticulospinal pathways), rubrospinal tracts (corticorubrospinal pathways), and vestibulospinal tracts.

sympathetic systems (see Chap. 17). These supraspinal fibers are often called the upper motor neurons of the autonomic nervous system.

Extrapyramidal System (Fig. 9.2)

The descending supraspinal tracts, their nuclei, and feedback circuits, influencing somatic motor activity of voluntary muscles with the exception of the pyramidal system, are incorporated into the so-called "extrapyramidal system" (see Chap. 21). The term is loosely used, and many authorities have discarded it. The descending tracts, which convey influences to the lower motor neurons, are actually neuronal links in pathway systems of complex circuitry involving the cerebral cortex, basal ganglia, thalamus, cerebellum, brainstem reticular formation, and related structures. Such systems include the corticorubrospinal, cerebellorubrospinal, corticoreticulospinal, cerebelloreticulospinal, cerebellovestibulospinal, and vestibular nerve–vestibulospinal pathways. The extrapyramidal system is discussed in Chap. 21.

Corticospinal (Pyramidal) Tract (Fig. 9.1)

The fibers of the *corticospinal tracts* originate in the cerebral cortex and descend through the ipsilateral posterior limb of the internal capsule (near genu), middle portion of the crus cerebri of midbrain, pons, and pyramids of the medulla. At the medulla–spinal cord junction, approximately 90 percent of the 1 million fibers in each tract cross as the pyramidal decussation and descend in the posterior half of the lateral funiculus as the non-somatotopically organized *lateral corticospinal tract,* which terminates at all spinal levels in laminae IV through VII and IX (see Chap. 5, "Spinal Cord in Cross Section"). About 8 percent of the fibers descend without crossing in the ipsilateral anterior funiculus as the anterior corticospinal tract, which terminates after crossing in the anterior white commissure in lamina VIII in the cervical and upper thoracic cord levels. A few pyramidal fibers descend as uncrossed axons in the lateral corticospinal tract.

The functional role of this pathway may be summarized as follows: (1) The fibers terminating in laminae IV and V are corticonuclear fibers which modulate and modify the sensory input of ascending sensory pathways— these descending fibers originate in the sensory cortex of the parietal lobe including the postcentral gyrus; (2) other fibers, terminating in the other laminae, interact with the interneurons of reflex circuits innervating the alpha and gamma motor neurons; and (3) some fibers terminating in lamina IX synapse directly with the lower motor neurons. In general, the corticospinal tracts facilitate flexor reflex activity. The numerous fibers terminating directly with lower motor neurons of lamina IX in the cervical (brachial) enlargement are functional correlates of the well-developed manipulative ability and digital dexterity of the human hand and fingers.

CORTICOBULBAR AND CORTICORETICULAR FIBERS

The *cortical (supranuclear, upper motor neuron)* projections to the nuclei of the *cranial nerves* and their ascending pathways comprise three types.

1 *Direct corticobulbar fibers* from each hemisphere to the motor nuclei of the cranial nerves originate in the cerebral cortex, descend in the genu of the internal capsule, and pass as crossed and uncrossed fibers to and through both the ipsilateral and contralateral brainstem before synapsing with the lower motor neurons of the motor nuclei of cranial nerves V (muscles of mastication), VII (muscles of facial expression), and XII (tongue musculature) (see Fig. 9.1). The lower motor neurons innervating the muscles of facial expression below the level of the eye (e.g., buccinator, labial muscles) are a clinically significant exception (see Chap. 14); they are innervated only by corticobulbar fibers which have decussated (not innervated by descending uncrossed fibers).

2 *Indirect corticobulbar fibers* (often included with the *corticoreticular fibers*) originate in the premotor, motor, and somesthetic areas of the cerebral cortex, descend in the genu of the internal capsule, and pass through both the ipsilateral and contralateral brainstem before synapsing with interneurons of the brainstem reticular formation (Fig. 9.1 and see *pseudobulbar palsy* in Chap. 14, "Basal Region of the Midbrain"). These interneurons are integrated in circuits which innervate the cranial nerve motor nuclei including ns. III, IV, V, VI, VII and XII and the nucleus ambiguus. The descending influences to the nucleus of the accessory nerve are probably conveyed via uncrossed indirect corticobulbar projections, which facilitate the contraction of the ipsilateral sternocleidomastoid and trapezius muscles.

3 *Corticonuclear fibers* project influences to nuclei of the ascending pathways including the nuclei gracilis and cuneatus of the posterior column–medial lemniscal pathway, principal sensory trigeminal nucleus, spinal trigeminal nucleus, and the nucleus of the solitary fasciculus. These fibers are involved with processing sensory influences in the nuclei of ascending pathways.

RETICULOSPINAL PATHWAYS

The *reticulospinal tracts* originate from cells in the medial two-thirds of the lower brainstem reticular formation (pons and medulla). No reticulospinal fibers originate in the midbrain. Through the corticoreticular fibers from the cerebral cortex, these tracts are integrated into the *corticoreticulospinal pathways* (Fig. 9.2). The *lateral (medullary)* reticulospinal tract and the *medial (pontine)* reticulospinal tract extend throughout the spinal cord, are not somatotopically organized, and exert influences through spinal interneurons on the alpha and gamma motor neurons.

The fibers of the lateral (medullary) reticulospinal tract originate from cells in the nucleus reticularis gigantocellularis of the medulla, descend mainly as uncrossed fibers in the anterior region of the lateral funiculus, and terminate at all spinal levels upon interneurons in lamina VII and adjacent areas of laminae VI and IX. This tract exerts inhibitory influences on extensor myotatic reflexes and muscle tone.

The fibers of the medial (pontine) reticulospinal tracts originate in the nucleus reticularis pontis caudalis and nucleus reticularis pontis oralis of the pontine reticular formation, descend mainly as uncrossed fibers in the anterior funiculus (included with medial longitudinal fasciculus, see below), and terminate at all spinal levels on interneurons in lamina VIII and the adjacent area of lamina VII. This tract exerts facilitatory influences on extensor motor neurons and muscle tone. The reticulospinal fibers convey impulses to spinal interneurons and their intrinsic spinal circuits on alpha and gamma motor neurons of reciprocally innervated muscle groups.

RUBROSPINAL TRACT

The fibers of the rubrospinal tract originate from cells located in the nucleus ruber, decussate immediately as the anterior tegmental decussation of the midbrain, descend through the brainstem tegmentum and lateral funiculus of the spinal cord, and terminate at all spinal levels with interneurons in the lateral portions of laminae V, VI, and VII (Fig. 9.2). This somatotopically organized tract exerts influences through intrinsic spinal circuits on the alpha and gamma motor neurons. The tract facilitates flexor motor tone (inhibits extensor muscle tone). The posterior and posteromedial regions of the nucleus ruber project to the cervical enlargement (upper extremity), whereas the anterior and anterolateral regions project to the lumbosacral enlargement (lower extremity). Most of the rubrospinal fibers terminate in the cervical spinal segments.

The nucleus ruber receives much of its input from the cerebral motor cortex via uncrossed *corticorubral fibers* and from the dentate and emboliform nuclei of the cerebellum via decussating *cerebellorubral fibers*. The corticorubrospinal fiber system is an indirect corticospinal pathway, with the red nucleus intercalated within the system; both systems relay influences from the cerebral motor cortex to the spinal cord (Fig. 9.2). The corticorubrospinal system seems to have an important functional role in skilled and dexterous movements.

VESTIBULOSPINAL TRACTS

The vestibular nuclei, located on the floor of the fourth ventricle of the upper medulla and lower pons, receive their input (1) via the vestibular nerve from the receptors of the membranous labyrinth (semicircular canals, utricle, and saccule), (2) from the vestibulocerebellum, and (3) from the fastigial nucleus of the cerebellum (see Fig. 15.4). Fibers from these vestibular nuclei project to some brainstem reticular nuclei, to certain cranial nerve nuclei (III, IV, and VI) via ascending fibers in the medial longitudinal fasciculus (see Fig. 13.3), and to the spinal cord via the *lateral* and the *medial vestibulospinal tracts*. There are no corticovestibular projections from the cerebral cortex.

Fibers from the lateral vestibular nucleus descend as the uncrossed, somatotopically organized lateral vestibulospinal tract in the anterior region of the lateral funiculus, and terminate upon interneurons in laminae VIII and adjacent VII of all levels of the spinal cord (Fig. 9.2). The anterorostral region of the lateral vestibular nucleus projects to the cervical enlargement, and the posterocaudal region to the lumbosacral enlargement. Functionally this tract influences muscle tone and postural movements by facilitating extensor muscle tone.

Fibers from the medial vestibular nucleus descend mainly as uncrossed fibers (medial vestibulospinal tract) within the medial longitudinal fasciculus of the anterior funiculus. They terminate upon neurons of laminae VIII and adjacent VII in the cervical and upper thoracic levels. The influences on muscle tone and posture are primarily inhibitory to extension activity.

MEDIAL LONGITUDINAL FASCICULUS

The *medial longitudinal fasciculus* (MLF) is a bundle of fibers in the brainstem (located anterior to the fourth ventricle and adjacent to the midline) and in the anterior funiculus of the cervical spinal cord. The MLF comprises the descending *tectospinal, interstitiospinal, medial vestibulospinal,* and *medial reticulospinal tracts;* it includes the ascending fibers from the vestibular nuclei in the pons and midbrain. The tectospinal fibers project from the superior colliculus, cross as the posterior tegmental decussation in the midbrain, and terminate in lamina VIII of the cervical levels. The tract is presumed to mediate reflexes responding to visual and possibly auditory stimuli. Some *tectobulbar (tectotegmental) fibers* project to the brainstem reticular nuclei, and are integrated into tectotegmentospinal pathways. The *interstitiospinal tract* from the interstitial nucleus of Cajal in the midbrain descends in the MLF and terminates in cervical levels; it has an unknown functional role. The medial vestibulospinal and medial reticulospinal tracts are described above. Fibers from the superior, medial, and lateral vestibular nuclei ascend as crossed and uncrossed fibers in the MLF to cranial nerve nuclei III, IV, and VI, innervating the extraocular muscles (see Fig. 13.3).

DESCENDING SOMATIC INFLUENCES

The descending pathways from the higher centers in the brain probably produce movements (1) by sending "direct" influences to the alpha motor neurons, and (2) by sending "indirect" influences to the gamma motor neurons and thereby acting through a feedback loop from the spindle to produce the desired contraction. Upon stimulation, the central nuclei in the brain have been shown to produce or to inhibit movement; hence the basic generalization that each central nucleus probably is able to excite (or to inhibit) the alpha and gamma motor neurons involved in the same basic contraction in much the same manner. In brief, both alpha and gamma motor nuclei are normally coinfluenced by descending pathways (this is called *"servo-assistance" of movement*). Thus in finger movements and respiratory movements, for example, the essential contraction of a muscle group through the alpha motor neurons commences just prior to the rise in the spindle firing from gamma stimulation. The latter has facilitated the essential contraction. Stated simply, the descending tracts from the brain convey influences which essentially bias the intrinsic activity of the spinal reflex circuitry.

In general usage, spinal reflexes are basically responses to neural influences conveyed as action potentials from the peripheral receptors. In contrast, voluntary activities are responses to neural influences conveyed as action potentials from the brain to the spinal cord. Voluntary activities need not be initiated by volitional drives. Under natural conditions neurons function in groups; thus a natural stimulus evokes many action potentials, called a volley, which influence the functional activity of a group of physiologically characterized neurons—called a neuronal pool. The inputs to a neuronal pool are expressed as excitatory and inhibitory postsynaptic potentials (EPSPs and IPSPs), whereas the output of reflex and voluntary activity via the lower motor neurons is expressed as obligatory excitatory responses of muscle contractions.

FIBERS OF THE AUTONOMIC NERVOUS SYSTEM

Influences from the hypothalamus, various cranial nerves, and other sources (see Chap. 18) are projected to the brainstem tegmentum where further processing occurs in the bilaterally organized reticuloreticular linkages of neurons within the brainstem reticular formation. The output from this region is conveyed (1) to the parasympathetic nuclei of cranial nerves III, VII, IX, and X located in the brainstem (see Chap. 17), and (2) via reticulospinal fibers descending within the anterolateral funiculus of the spinal cord to lamina VII. Influences from the latter are projected to the intermediolateral cell column in the thoracic and upper lumbar levels (T1 through L2)—the outflow of the sympathetic nervous system—and to the midsacral levels (S2 through S4)—the outflow of the parasympathetic nervous system (see Chap. 17). Within the lower brainstem reticular formation are functionally defined regions called *respiratory centers* and *cardiovascular centers*. These centers affect the expiratory and inspiratory phases of respiration and exert pressor and depressor effects on the circulatory system.

Chapter 10

Lesions of the Spinal Nerves and Spinal Cord

Injuries to the nervous system and neurologic diseases produce symptoms and clinical signs. The following outline is presented for its value in reinforcing an understanding of the normal anatomy and physiology of the spinal cord.

LESIONS OF THE VENTRAL ROOTS

Depending on the specific spinal level, lesions of the ventral roots interrupt specific alpha and gamma motor neurons and preganglionic autonomic fibers (Fig. 10.1, No. 1). The injury of all the lower motor neurons innervating a muscle or group of muscles results in a lower motor neuron paralysis or paresis of that muscle or muscles. This occurs in poliomyelitis—the polio virus may selectively affect lower motor neurons of the spinal cord and of the brainstem. When the preganglionic autonomic fibers are injured, trophic effects may accompany the lower motor neuron paralysis (see below).

Lower Motor Neuron Paralysis

The signs of a *lower motor neuron (flaccid) paralysis* and associated trophic changes include the following:

77

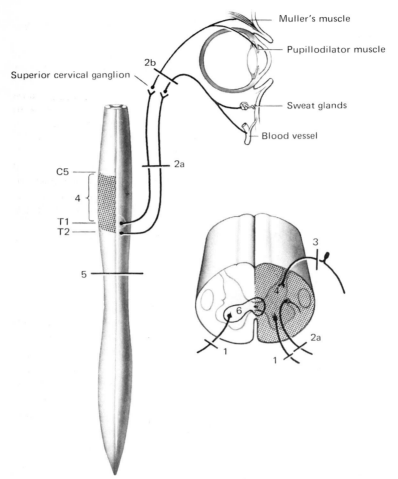

Figure 10.1 Schemata of the spinal cord to indicate the site of lesions noted in the text. The arabic numbers refer to specific lesions. C5 to T1 indicate the cervical enlargement, the region involved with the innervation of the upper extremity. 1, ventral roots of spinal nerves; 2a, preganglionic sympathetic fibers from T1 to T2 levels; 2b, postganglionic sympathetic fibers from the superior cervical ganglion; 3, dorsal roots of spinal nerves; 4, hemisection of the spinal cord (Brown-Séquard syndrome) extending through the cervical enlargement; 5, transection of the spinal cord at a midthoracic level; and 6, lesion in region surrounding central canal throughout the cervical enlargement and extending into the anterior horn at the C8 and T1 level on one side.

1 All voluntary movements are abolished, and reflex contractions cannot be elicited when all the lower motor neurons innervating a group of muscles are interrupted. The muscles are paralyzed. A *paresis* (*partial paralysis*) results when some, but not all, of the lower motor neurons normally innervating the muscle are functional.

2   The paralyzed muscles are flaccid, offer no resistance to passive movement, and have lost their tone (*atony*). Because the myotatic reflex arcs are not intact, the *deep tendon reflexes* (*DTRs*) are absent (*areflexia*). If some of the lower motor neurons are functional, the tonus is reduced (*hypotonus*), and the DTRs are weak (*hyporeflexia*).

3   Reaching a peak about 2 to 3 weeks following denervation, muscles spontaneously contract. In time, the muscles atrophy. The spontaneous contractions of muscle fibers are known as fibrillations and fasciculations. They are expressions of trophic changes. Fibrillation is a single muscle-fiber contraction, which can only be seen when the affected muscle is thinly covered as in the tongue and, rarely, in the hand. It is a response associated with the hypersensitivity of a denervated muscle (Chap. 17). Fasciculations are the muscle twitchings visible through the skin resulting from the spontaneous discharge of motor units. As lower motor neurons die, they discharge repetitively to produce fasciculations of the muscles they innervate.

4   The trophic changes include a dry, cyanotic skin which may be ulcerated (see below).

Trophic Functions and Changes

In addition to stimulating muscles to contract and glands to secrete, the nervous system exerts effects that initiate and regulate the molecular organization of other cells. These effects are expressions of the *trophic* (literally *nutritional*) functions of the nervous system. Trophic changes include the alterations that occur after lesions of the fibers of the autonomic nervous system in the central or the peripheral nervous system. Among these disturbances are a dry, warm or cool, flushed or cyanotic skin (change in capillary circulation), abnormal brittleness of fingernails, loss of hair, dryness or ulcerations of the skin, and lysis of the bones and joints.

Such *trophic effects* (*trophic influences*) of neurons are directed to different types of target tissues, including epithelium, nerve endings (e.g., taste buds), and muscle cells.

Transection of Sympathetic Fibers to the Head

Lesion of preganglionic sympathetic fibers in the ventral roots of T1 and T2, the cervical sympathetic trunk, or of the postganglionic sympathetic neurons of the superior cervical ganglion (see Chap. 17) will result in *Horner's syndrome* on the ipsilateral side of the face (Fig. 10.1, No. 2a and b). The affected pupil is smaller than the pupil of the opposite eye; it does not dilate when the pupil is shaded (pupillodilator muscle unit is not stimulated to contract). The affected eyelid droops a bit (ptosis) because the superior palpebral smooth muscle (Muller's muscle) is denervated. The face is dry (denervated sweat glands), red, and warm (vasodilatation of cutaneous blood vessels).

LESIONS OF THE DORSAL ROOTS

The irritation of the fibers of one dorsal root (radix) by mechanical compression (tumor or slipped disk) or a local inflammation may produce pain with a radicular distribution (Fig. 10.1, No. 3). Because adjacent dermatomes overlap, the destruction of one dorsal root (e.g., by transection) may result in the slight diminution of all sensations (*hypesthesia*) in part of the dermatome innervated by that dorsal root. Destruction of several consecutive dorsal roots does result in the complete absence of all sensations (*anesthesia*) in all but the rostral and caudal dermatomes innervated by the sectioned roots. Irritation to the dorsal root fibers may result in *paresthesia* (abnormal spontaneous sensations such as numbness and prickling) or *hyperesthesia* (excessive sensibility to sensory stimuli in pain). The stimulation of a dorsal root may result in a *dermatomal vasodilatation* (due to reflex arc involving the autonomic nervous system).

If all dorsal roots innervating the upper extremity (C5 through T1) are transected (e.g., surgically by dorsal root rhizotomy), several symptoms may be additionally observed. Because the afferent limb of the reflex arcs is interrupted, reflex activity is absent (areflexia), and muscles are hypotonic. Although the limb muscles are not paralyzed (lower motor neurons are intact), motor activity is impaired. The deafferented limb hangs by the side and is generally not used. It can be volitionally moved when facilitatory influences from the descending supraspinal motor pathways stimulate the lower motor neurons.

Lesions and irritations of the dorsal roots or posterior horn result in segmental (dermatomal) sensory disturbances. In dorsal root lesions all general senses in the region innervated by the root fibers (dermatome) are lost or diminished. In posterior horn lesions a *dissociated sensory loss* (loss of one sensation and the preservation of others) may occur in the dermatome, with, for example, pain and temperature sensibilities lost or reduced, but touch and other associated general senses intact and normal. Dissociated sensory loss of pain and temperature also occurs in lesions in the vicinity of the central canal (see "Syringomyelia" below).

LESIONS OF THE UPPER MOTOR NEURONS;
UPPER MOTOR NEURON PARALYSIS

Interruption of the upper motor neurons (pyramidal tract and other descending supraspinal tracts) results in motor disturbances known as an *upper motor neuron paralysis*. Clinically, this paralysis is generally attributed to lesions of the pyramidal tract. Immediately after the occurrence of the lesion, the deep tendon reflexes are temporarily depressed and the paralysed muscles are flaccid. In time, weeks and months later, the muscles become spastic, that is, there is increased muscle tone (hypertonus), increased deep tendon reflexes (hyperreflexia), and clonus. Hence an upper motor neuron paralysis is called a *spastic paralysis.* Such a paralysis of the upper and lower extremities on one side is called a *hemiplegia.*

1   Hypertonus is expressed in the firmness and stiffness of muscles— primarily in the flexors of the upper extremities and in the extensors of the lower extremities. These are antigravity muscles—the upper limb holds itself up and the lower limb supports the body. The brisk knee jerk following the tapping of the quadriceps tendon is an example of hyperreflexia. With the passive movement of the spastic body part, muscular resistance increases, especially in the extensors of the lower extremities and the flexors of the upper extremities. The spastic signs of an upper motor neuron paralysis may be due primarily to an increased activity of the dynamic fusiform system (Chap. 5). At the beginning of a movement, the resistance is strong, but it soon yields suddenly, as force against the resistance is maintained, in a clasp-knife (jackknife) fashion. The sudden yielding of resistance is due to the surge of inhibitory influences from the activity of the Golgi tendon organs of the stretched tendons (called the *inverse myotatic reflex*).

2   *Clonus* is the rhythmic oscillation of a joint (e.g., ankle or knee) which occurs when a second party suddenly dorsiflexes the foot (pressure on the sole of foot pushes toes toward knee) and maintains the dorsiflexion attitude under elastic pressure. The dorsiflexion actually puts the gastrocnemius muscle and its Achilles tendon under moderate stretch. Clonus persists as long as the muscle is kept in this state of stretch.

3   There is also loss or diminution of cutaneous or superficial reflexes. Stimulation of the skin of the thorax, abdomen, or extremities evoke weak or no reflex responses.

4   The *Babinski reflex* (sign) can be elicited. When the lateral aspect of the sole of the foot is stroked with a blunt point, the big toe dorsiflexes (hyperextension), the tip of the toe points to the knee, and the other toes spread (fan).

SPINAL CORD HEMISECTION (BROWN-SÉQUARD SYNDROME)

A hemisection (unilateral transverse lesion) of the spinal cord damages structures, which results in a number of changes in the body at, and below, the levels caudal to the lesion (Fig. 10.1, No. 4). For instructional purposes, assume that the lesion is a hemisection extending from C5 through T1 spinal levels; the peripheral nerves associated with these spinal levels innervate the upper extremity.

In relating the side of a lesion (right or left) in the nervous system to the side of the body where signs are expressed, one must relate the site of the pathway's crossing over to the location of the lesion. Symptoms occur on the same side (ipsilateral) and below the level of the lesion when the damaged neurons are those which normally convey influences from the same side of the body (ascending sensory tract) or to the same side of the body (descending motor tracts). In the spinal cord, structures involved with ipsilateral functional roles include the posterior columns, dorsal roots, lateral corticospinal tract (and other upper motor neurons), and ventral roots. Symptoms occur on the opposite (contralateral) side below the level of the lesion when the damaged neurons convey information from or to the opposite side of the body. In the spinal cord, this includes the decussated fibers of the lateral and anterior spinothalamic tract. In the brainstem this includes the spinothalamic tract, medial lemniscus, and corticospinal tract.

The fiber tracts injured and resultant symptoms and signs include:

1 Posterior column (fasciculi gracilis and cuneatus). Loss of position sense, appreciation of passive movement, vibratory sense, and two-point discrimination on the same side at and below the spinal levels of the lesion. The modalities from the neck are unaffected because the fibers conveying them are located wholly above the level of the lesion.

2 Lateral spinothalamic tract. Loss of pain and temperature on the opposite side at and below the spinal levels of the lesion. This includes the contralateral upper extremity because lateral spinothalamic fibers decussate within one or two levels of the spinal root origin.

3 Anterior spinothalamic tract. Tactile sensibility is probably little affected on the opposite side below the spinal level of the lesion because this modality is also conveyed in the uncrossed fasciculi gracilis and cuneatus.

4 Corticospinal tracts and other descending supraspinal tracts. The spastic syndrome following the interruption of these fibers results in an upper motor neuron paralysis including spasticity, hyperactive deep tendon reflexes (*DTRs, hyperreflexia*), diminution or loss of superficial reflexes, Babinski sign, and muscle clonus below (but not at level of) the site of lesion on the ipsilateral side. The hyperactive DTRs are illustrated by a brisk knee jerk or ankle jerk.

5 At the spinal levels of the transection (C5 through T1), the entering fibers of the dorsal roots and the emerging fibers of the lower motor neurons and preganglionic sympathetic fibers (C8 and T1) are interrupted. The result is the complete absence of all sensations in the upper extremity on the side of lesion. Pain and temperature are lost on the contralateral upper extremity due to the lesion of the lateral spinothalamic tract on the side of lesion. Paresthesias and radicular pain may be sensed over the ipsilateral C5 and T1 dermatomes from the irritation of some intact dorsal root fibers; because of dermatome overlap from C4 and T2, the C5 and T1 dermatomes have a hypesthesia. The entire ipsilateral limb is flaccid; it exhibits all the signs of a lower motor neuron paralysis. Horner's syndrome on the ipsilateral side of the face and trophic changes in the ipsilateral upper extremity are due to the interruption of the preganglionic sympathetic neurons (see Chap. 17).

SPINAL CORD TRANSECTION (PARAPLEGIA)

Immediately after the complete transection of the spinal cord (Fig. 10.1, No. 5), the nervous system caudal to the lesion site is devoid of detectable neural activity. All voluntary movements and somatic and visceral reflex activities are abolished. Sensibilities from the body below the transection level are absent. This period of extremely depressed activity called *spinal shock* lasts about 2 to 3 weeks in man (it varies in duration from 4 days to 6 weeks). Spinal shock is apparently due to the sudden withdrawal of influences from the descending pathways, especially the corticospinal tract.

The isolated spinal cord and its spinal nerves gradually exhibit autonomous neural activity which is divided into a sequence of phases of variable lengths: (1) minimal reflex activity, (2) flexor spasm activity (superficial reflexes), (3) alternation between flexor and extensor spasm activities, and (4) predominant extensor spasm activity (deep reflexes). After a year or two, paraplegic patients may be placed in one of several categories: (1) that in which extensor spasms predominate over flexor spasms, called *paraplegia-in-extension* (observed in about two-thirds of paraplegics); (2) that in which flexor spasms predominate, called *paraplegia-in-flexion;* and (3) that in which a flaccid paralysis persists (less than 20 percent). The absence of autonomic nervous system influences from the brain is accompanied by a variety of disturbances in the control of automatic activities of the urinary, genital, and anorectal systems.

SYRINGOMYELIA

A syrinx (cavity) may develop in the region of the central canal of the cervical enlargement; from there the gliosis and cavitation may extend to other sites (Fig. 10.1, No. 6). The initial clinical signs are the loss of pain and temperature sensibility with a bilateral segmental distribution in both upper extremities. This dissociated sensory loss is due to the interruption of the decussating lateral spinothalamic fibers in the anterior white commissure. There is no sensory loss in the body and lower extremities because the spinothalamic tracts and dorsal columns are intact. The extension of the degeneration into the anterior horns of C8 and T1 on one side produces, on the side of the lesion, lower motor neuron disturbances and trophic changes on the ulnar side of the arm and forearm and the fourth and fifth fingers, and possibly Horner's syndrome.

TABES DORSALIS

Tabes dorsalis is a form of neurosyphilis in which the primary pathology of the dorsal root ganglia is accompanied by degenerative changes in the posterior columns, especially in the fasciculi gracilis bilaterally. The pain fibers are also involved. In the initial stages, the irritation of dorsal root fibers produces paresthesias and intermittent attacks of sharp pain. In time, the symptoms include diminished sensitivity to pain; loss of kinesthetic sense; diminished-to-absent deep tendon reflexes (ankle and knee jerks); loss of muscle tone; and marked impairment of muscle, joint, and vibratory senses accompanied by an ataxic gait. Patients walk with legs held apart, head bent, and eyes looking down, raising their knees high and slapping their feet on the ground. The eyes stare at the ground to pick up cues which substitute for the lost kinesthetic senses.

AMYOTROPHIC LATERAL SCLEROSIS

Amyotrophic lateral sclerosis is a degenerative motor tract disease with bilateral involvement of the pyramidal tracts and anterior horns. Because there is degeneration of both upper and lower motor neurons, signs of both upper and lower motor neuron paralysis are expressed. Most of the affected muscles show evidence of the degeneration of lower motor neurons, including paralysis, atrophy, fasciculations, and weakness; these signs are initially expressed by the muscles of the hands and arms. Some muscles exhibit signs of upper motor neuron paralysis, hyperreflexia, and, at times, Babinski signs. The lower motor neurons of cranial nerves may also exhibit signs of degeneration.

COMBINED SYSTEM DEGENERATION

Combined system degeneration is a complication of pernicious anemia (a disease due to lack of intrinsic factor for absorption of vitamin B_{12}) in which there is subacute degeneration bilaterally of the fibers of the posterior columns and lateral columns, especially those involved with the lumbosacral cord. The clinical symptoms include: (1) loss of position and vibratory senses, numbness, and dysesthesias in the lower extremities, and (2) such upper motor neuron signs as spasticity, muscle weakness, hyperactive deep tendon reflexes, and Babinski reflexes.

DEGENERATION, REGENERATION, AND SPROUTING

An injured neuron reacts to an insult, whether it is a transection, a crush, a toxic substance, or a deprivation of blood supply. The entire neuron responds and may reconstitute itself.

Degeneration

The degenerative reactions following transection include changes in (1) the cell body (chromatolysis), (2) the nerve fiber between the cell body and the trauma (primary degeneration), and (3) the nerve fiber distal to the trauma (secondary or Wallerian degeneration). The cell body swells, Nissl bodies undergo "dissolution" or chromatolysis, and the nucleus is displaced to the side of the cell body. These are manifestations of metabolic activities which can ultimately lead to the regeneration of the severed fiber. The chromatolysis is indicative of the enhanced protein synthesis. The few degenerative changes in the nerve proximal to the cut include the breakdown of the myelin sheath and axon in the vicinity of the injury. The axon and myelin sheath of the fiber distal to the trauma become fragmented and are removed by macrophages (this takes place usually over a period of weeks).

Terminal Regeneration

Regeneration is essentially a process of differentiation and growth. The neurolemma (Schwann) cells in the proximal stump near the trauma and in the distal stump divide mitotically to form continuous cords of neurolemma cells. These cords extend from the proximal stump, through the small gap between the stumps into the distal stump, and up to the sites of the sensory receptors and motor endings. The cell bodies synthesize proteins and other metabolites which flow distally into the regenerating and lengthening axons. The terminal ends (terminal regeneration) of the proximal axons branch into numerous sprouts which grow distally at an optimal rate of 4 mm per day into the gap and distal stump along the neurolemmal cords (act as guidelines) to the sites of the nerve endings. Each regenerating axon of the proximal stump may divide to form as many as 50 terminal sprouts. In turn, each neurolemmal cord may act as the guiding scaffold for numerous regenerating axons. The surviving regenerating axons are those that terminate in the proper nerve endings. The potential of each neurolemmal cord to act as a guide for many regenerating axons increases the possibility of reinnervating the receptor associated with its cord. When fully myelinated, each regenerating branch tends to have a conduction velocity of about 80 percent of that of the original fiber. The superfluous axonal branches eventually degenerate.

Collateral Sprouting

A denervated neurolemmal cord is presumed to exert trophic influences upon a nearby normal nerve fiber; the latter responds by sprouting new collateral branches from its nodes of Ranvier. This is known as *preterminal axonal sprouting* or *collateral nerve sprouting*. The collateral branch joins the axonless neurolemmal cord, grows down the cord, and reinnervates the nerve ending. Collateral nerve sprouting occurs in both the peripheral nervous system and central nervous system (the latter does not have neurolemmal cords).

Chapter 11

Brainstem: Medulla, Pons, and Midbrain

GENERAL ORGANIZATION

The infratentorial *brainstem* comprises the medulla, pons, and midbrain (Figs. 1.2, 1.4, and 11.1 through 11.3). The diencephalon is the supratentorial brainstem. The brainstem is anatomically organized as four structures oriented parallel to the neuraxis: roof, ventricular cavity, tegmentum, and basilar portion.

The posteriorly located roof is called the tectum (quadrigeminal plate) in the midbrain, cerebellum in the pons, and the tela choroidea and its choroid plexus in the medulla. Although the cerebellum is technically not a brainstem structure, the cerebellum and the functionally unimportant velum form the pontine roof (Fig. 1.2). The *ventricular cavity* includes the cerebral aqueduct (iter) in the midbrain and the fourth ventricle in the pons and medulla (Figs. 11.4 and 11.5). The tegmentum is called the tegmentum throughout the length of the brainstem. The anteriorly located basilar portion is called the crus cerebri in the midbrain, ventral portion or pons proper in the pons, and the pyramids in the medulla (Figs. 11.4 and 11.5).

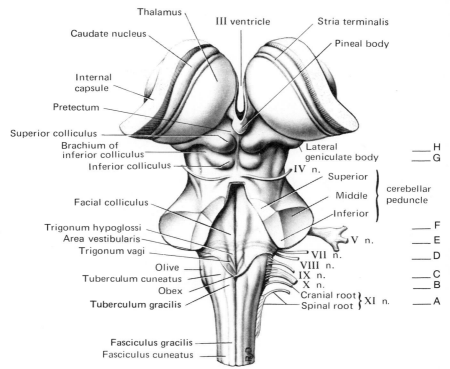

Figure 11.1 Posterior surface of the brainstem. The lines adjacent to the letters indicate the levels of the transverse sections illustrated in Figs. 11.4 and 11.5. Roman numerals represent some cranial nerves (Chap. 12). For explanation of A to H, see text.

The midbrain *tectum* includes the pretectum (light reflex, Chap. 16), superior colliculus (optic reflexes, Chap. 16), inferior colliculus (auditory system, Chap. 13), and the emerging trochlear nerve (n. IV) caudally.

The *tegmentum* is composed of (1) cranial nerve nuclei and portions of their nerve fibers, (2) ascending pathways, (3) descending pathways, and (4) the reticular formation. Emerging from the lateral surface of the brainstem are cranial nerves V, VII, VIII, IX, X, and XI (Figs. 12.1 and 12.2). Emerging on the anterior surface of the brainstem are cranial nerves III, VI, and XII. The *reticular formation* contains the ascending and descending reticular pathways and reticular nuclei. Some of the reticular nuclei are the nucleus reticularis gigantocellularis, inferior olivary nucleus, and lateral reticular nucleus of the medulla; nuclei reticularis pontis caudalis and oralis of the pons; red nucleus (nucleus rubrum) and substantia nigra of the midbrain. The substantia nigra may be included in the basilar portion.

The *basilar portion* consists of descending pathways from the cerebral

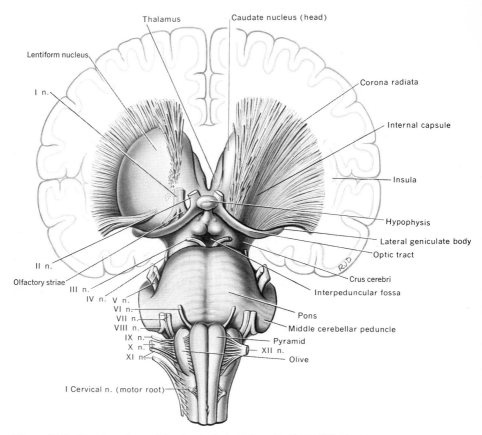

Figure 11.2 Basal surface of the brainstem and roots of cranial nerves.

cortex. These include (1) the corticobulbar and corticoreticular fibers which terminate in the brainstem tegmentum, and the corticospinal tract which terminates in the spinal cord (Figs. 9.1 and 9.2), and (2) the corticopontine (to pontine nuclei of pons proper) and pontocerebellar fibers (see Chap. 15).

FUNCTIONAL ELEMENTS OF THE BRAINSTEM

Conceptually the structural organization of the functional elements of the brainstem can be visualized by understanding the location, topography, and orientation of several structures, namely: (1) cranial nerves and their nuclei, (2) ascending lemniscal pathways, (3) reticular formation: its nuclei and pathways, (4) descending pathways, and (5) pathways to and from the cerebellum (see Chap. 15).

not responsible

CRANIAL NERVES AND THEIR NUCLEI
(See Also Chap. 12)

end of chapter

Afferent Sensory Fibers and Their Nuclei of Termination (Fig. 12.1)

The sensory cranial nerves (ns.) with *general somatic afferent* (*GSA*), *general visceral afferent* (*GVA*), and/or *special visceral afferent* (*SVA*) fibers, are (1) the trigeminal nerve V with GSA fibers, and (2) the facial nerve VII, glossopharyngeal nerve IX, and vagus nerve X, each with GSA, GVA, and SVA fibers. The neurons of the first order of each of these nerves are located in sensory ganglia that are the equivalents of the dorsal root ganglia of spinal nerves. They are the trigeminal (Gasserian, semilunar) ganglion of n. V, the geniculate ganglion of n. VII, and the superior and inferior ganglia each of ns. IX and X. The GSA fibers of each of these nerves terminate in the principal (chief, main) sensory nucleus of n. V (located in the pons) or descend in the spinal trigeminal tract before terminating in the spinal trigeminal nucleus located in the lateral lower pons and medulla and substantia gelatinosa of the first two cervical spinal segments. The GVA and SVA fibers descend in the solitary tract and terminate in the solitary nucleus located in the posterior medullary tegmentum. Some GSA fibers of n. V and other nerves have cell bodies in the mesencephalic nucleus of n. V located in the midbrain.

(*Text continues on p. 94*)

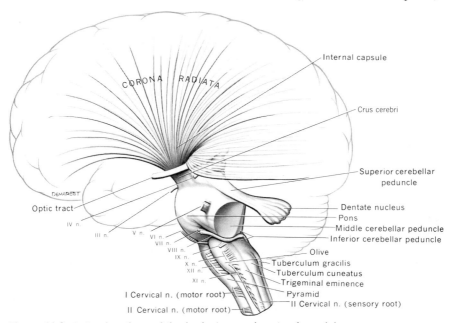

Figure 11.3 Lateral surface of the brainstem and roots of cranial nerves.

GUIDE TO FIGS. 11.4 AND 11.5

The internal anatomy of the brainstem can be more easily visualized once one understands the topographic relations of several tracts and cranial nerves.

1 In the lateral tegmentum, note the spinothalamic tract, anterior and posterior spinocerebellar tracts, spinal trigeminal tract, and the lateral lemniscus–brachium of the inferior colliculus auditory pathways.

2 In the anterior brainstem (basilar region), note the corticospinal and corticopontine tracts.

3 Just anterior to the central canal (cerebral aqueduct and fourth ventricle) on either side of the midline, note the medial longitudinal fasciculi.

4 Note that the medial lemniscus gradually shifts laterally and posteriorly as it ascends rostrally in the tegmentum from an anteromedial location in the medulla to a posterolateral location in the upper midbrain.

5 Note that cranial ns. III, VI, and XII emerge anteriorly from the brainstem; n. IV emerges posteriorly; and ns. V, VII, VIII, IX, X, and XI emerge laterally from the brainstem.

Fig. 11.4

Section D Note (1) the large fourth ventricle roofed posteriorly by the choroid plexus, (2) the large inferior olivary nuclei in the anterior tegmentum, (3) the motor cranial nerve nuclei (hypoglossal nucleus, dorsal vagal nucleus, and nucleus ambiguus) located medial to the sensory cranial nerve nuclei (nucleus solitarius and spinal nucleus of n. V), and (4) the laterally emerging vagus nerve and the anteriorly emerging hypoglossal nerve.

Section C Note the course of the internal arcuate fibers from the nuclei gracilis and cuneatus (located posteriorly) as they form an arc through the medullary tegmentum, decussate, and become the ascending medial lemniscus located in the anterior medial tegmentum.

Section B Note (1) the basic similarity to the spinal cord, (2) the presence of the nucleus gracilis in the posterior columns, and (3) the decussating fibers of the corticospinal tracts passing from the medullary pyramids (located anteromedially to the lateral white columns).

Section A Note the basic similarity to the composite section through the spinal cord (Fig. 5.3). The spinal trigeminal tract and nucleus are the rostral equivalents to the posterolateral tract of Lissauer and the substantia gelatinosa (lamina II), respectively. The lateral corticospinal tracts are located posteriorly in the lateral white columns.

Fig. 11.5

Section H   Note (1) the superior colliculus (Chap. 16), (2) n. III passing from the nucleus of n. III and emerging anteriorly, (3) the nucleus ruber associated with decussated fibers of the superior cerebellar peduncle (Chap. 15), and (4) the crus cerebri, which contains the corticospinal, corticobulbar, and corticopontine tracts.

Section G   Note (1) the medial lemniscus, spinothalamic tract, and lateral lemniscus, which have shifted laterally and posteriorly along the margin of the tegmentum, and (2) n. IV as it forms an arc along the periventricular gray before emerging from the tectum (actually the nerve emerges from the tectum at a level caudal to the nucleus of n. IV).

Section F   Note (1) the medial lemniscus, spinothalamic tract, and lateral lemniscus on the anterior and anterolateral aspects of the tegmentum, (2) the motor nucleus of n. V, which is medial to the principal sensory nucleus of n. V (n. V passes through the middle cerebellar peduncle before emerging from the lateral side of the brainstem), and (3) the middle and superior cerebellar peduncles (Chaps. 8 and 15).

Section E   Note (1) the auditory pathways including the cochlear nerve and nuclei, fibers of the trapezoid body, and the lateral lemniscus (Chap. 13), (2) the VIth nucleus and nerve (the nerve is incomplete in this diagram because the nerve emerges caudal to this level at the junction of the pons and the medulla), (3) n. VII, which emerges from its nucleus, passes postero-medially to, and hooks around the VIth nerve nucleus and courses antero-laterally before emerging from the brainstem laterally, (4) pontine nuclei (Chap. 15), and (5) inferior cerebellar peduncle (Chaps. 8, 13, and 15).

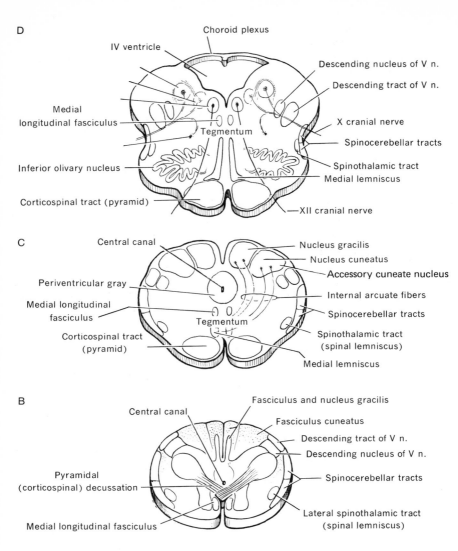

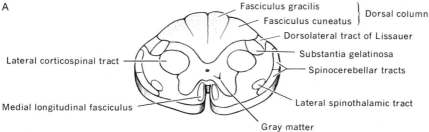

Figure 11.4 Transverse sections of spinal cord and medulla through (A) the upper first cervical segment of spinal cord, (B) the lower medulla at the level of the pyramidal (corticospinal) decussation, (C) the lower medulla at the level of the decussation of the medial lemniscus (internal arcuate fibers), and (D) midmedulla at the level of the middle of the inferior olivary nucleus. Sections correspond to levels indicated on Fig. 11.1.

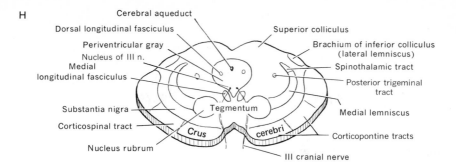

H

Cerebral aqueduct

Dorsal longitudinal fasciculus

Superior colliculus

Periventricular gray

Brachium of inferior colliculus
(lateral lemniscus)

Nucleus of III n.

Spinothalamic tract

Medial
longitudinal fasciculus

Posterior trigeminal
tract

Substantia nigra

Tegmentum

Medial lemniscus

Corticospinal tract

Crus   cerebri

Corticopontine tracts

Nucleus rubrum

III cranial nerve

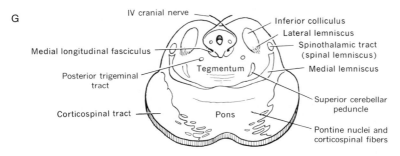

G

IV cranial nerve

Inferior colliculus

Lateral lemniscus

Medial longitudinal fasciculus

Spinothalamic tract
(spinal lemniscus)

Posterior trigeminal
tract

Tegmentum

Medial lemniscus

Corticospinal tract

Pons

Superior cerebellar
peduncle

Pontine nuclei and
corticospinal fibers

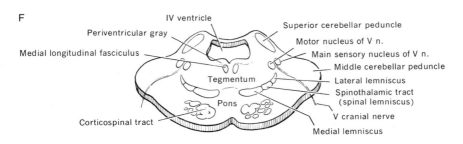

F

IV ventricle

Periventricular gray

Superior cerebellar peduncle

Motor nucleus of V n.

Medial longitudinal fasciculus

Main sensory nucleus of V n.

Middle cerebellar peduncle

Tegmentum

Lateral lemniscus

Spinothalamic tract
(spinal lemniscus)

Pons

V cranial nerve

Corticospinal tract

Medial lemniscus

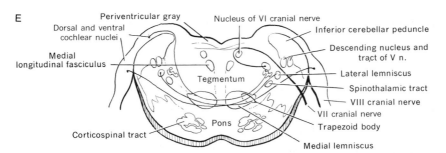

E

Periventricular gray

Nucleus of VI cranial nerve

Dorsal and ventral
cochlear nuclei

Inferior cerebellar peduncle

Descending nucleus and
tract of V n.

Medial
longitudinal fasciculus

Tegmentum

Lateral lemniscus

Spinothalamic tract

VIII cranial nerve

VII cranial nerve

Pons

Trapezoid body

Corticospinal tract

Medial lemniscus

Figure 11.5 Transverse sections of the pons and midbrain through (E) the lower pons at the level of the abducent, facial, and cochlear nerves, (F) the midpons at the level of the entrance of the Vth cranial nerve, (G) the lower midbrain at the level of the inferior colliculus, and (H) the upper midbrain at the level of the superior colliculus. Sections correspond to levels indicated on Fig. 11.1.

The *special somatic afferent* (*SSA*) fibers from the vestibular and cochlear receptors of the inner ear form the vestibular nerve and cochlear nerve (vestibulocochlear nerve). The fibers of these first-order neurons with their cell bodies in the vestibular and spiral ganglia enter on the posterolateral aspects of the upper pons before terminating in the vestibular nuclei and cerebellum (vestibular fibers) and the cochlear nuclei (cochlear fibers).

Motor Nuclei and Fibers of the Lower Motor Neurons of the Cranial Nerves (Fig. 12.2)

The *general somatic motor neurons* (*GSE;* lower motor neurons) have their cell bodies in the motor nuclei of n. III of the midbrain, n. IV of the lower midbrain, n. VI of the pons-medulla junction, and n. XII of the medulla. These nuclei are located in the tegmentum just ventral to the iter and fourth ventricle and on either side of the midline. The axons of these lower motor neurons emerge on the anterior brain surface just lateral to the midline (as the exception, n. IV emerges on the posterior surface of the lower midbrain). These nuclei and nerves are the cranial equivalents of the anterior horn cells (lamina IX) and ventral motor roots, respectively, of the spinal cord.

The *general visceral motor neurons* (*GVE,* preganglionic parasympathetic neurons of the autonomic nervous system; Chap. 17) have their cell bodies in the accessory oculomotor nucleus of Edinger-Westphal of n. III, in the superior and inferior salivatory nuclei, and in the dorsal vagal nucleus. The axons originating from the accessory oculomotor nucleus of Edinger-Westphal join n. III; those from the superior and inferior salivatory nuclei join ns. VII and IX, respectively; and those from the dorsal vagal nucleus join n. X. These neurons are the equivalents of the spinal preganglionic neurons of the spinal cord.

The *special visceral motor neurons of the branchiomeric nerves* (*SVE,* lower motor neurons) have their cell bodies in the motor nucleus of n. V of the midpons, in the motor nucleus of n. VII (facial nucleus) of the lower pons, and in the nucleus ambiguus of the medulla. All are located in the lateral tegmentum. The axons of the nucleus ambiguus join ns. IX, X, and XI. These neurons, all of which innervate the voluntary muscles of the branchiomeric arches, have no equivalent in the spinal cord except for the spinal component of n. XI.

ASCENDING PATHWAYS WITHIN THE BRAINSTEM

The ascending pathways in the brainstem include those that convey information from spinal cord and brainstem levels to the higher centers in the cerebrum and cerebellum. The ascending systems from spinal levels include the (1) posterior column–medial lemniscus system, (2) lateral and anterior spinothalamic tracts, (3) spinocervicothalamic pathway, (4) spinoreticular tract, and (5) spinocerebellar tracts (all are outlined in Chaps. 6 to 8). Additional ascending systems originating from brainstem levels include the (1) anterior and posterior trigeminothalamic tracts (general senses), (2) solitariothalamic tract (taste), (3) lateral lemniscus (audition), (4) medial longitudinal fasciculus (vestibular system), and (5) central tegmental tract of the reticular formation.

From Spinal Levels

The *medial lemniscus* of the posterior column–medial lemniscal pathway is a prominent, functionally significant, landmark within the brainstem (Fig. 7.1). From cell bodies in the nuclei gracilis and cuneatus, axons arc anteriorly and medially as the internal arcuate fibers which decussate and ascend as the medial lemniscus through the brainstem before terminating in the ventral posterolateral nucleus of the thalamus. In its ascent the medial lemniscus gradually shifts from its anteromedial location in the medulla (posterior to the pyramid), to the anterior tegmentum in the pons, and then to the posterolateral tegmentum in the midbrain.

The *lateral spinothalamic tract* (called *spinothalamic tract* or *spinal lemniscus* in the brainstem) ascends through the lateral tegmentum of the medulla and pons and in the posterolateral tegmentum of the midbrain before terminating in the ventral posterolateral nucleus and posterior thalamic region (Fig. 6.1). The fibers of the *anterior spinothalamic tract* ascend close to the spinothalamic tract in the brainstem (Fig. 7.1). The fibers of the spinocervicothalamic pathways (Fig. 8.1), which have recently been described in primates, probably pass through the brainstem close to the medial lemniscus.

The *spinoreticular fibers* and collateral branches of the lateral spinothalamic fibers terminate in the reticular formation (nucleus reticularis gigantocellularis and lateral reticular nucleus).

The *spinocerebellar pathways* are located in the lateral tegmentum of the brainstem (Fig. 8.1). The posterior spinocerebellar tract and the cuneocerebellar tract from the accessory cuneate nucleus pass through the inferior cerebellar peduncle and terminate in the paleocerebellum. The anterior spinocerebellar tract ascends to the midbrain, passes through the superior cerebellar peduncle, and terminates in the paleocerebellum. Fibers from the lateral reticular nucleus (receives input from spinal cord) project via inferior cerebellar peduncle to paleocerebellum.

From Brainstem Levels

Pain and temperature sensations from the face, forehead, and nasal and oral cavities are conveyed from the neurons in the spinal trigeminal nucleus via the *anterior trigeminal tract* (Fig. 6.1), which ascends as a crossed tract between the medial lemniscus and spinothalamic tract (Chap. 6). Other pain fiber projections from this nucleus are conveyed via the *trigeminoreticulo-thalamic pathway* (Fig. 6.1) in the brainstem reticular formation. The general discriminatory senses are relayed from the principal sensory nucleus of the trigeminal nerve via (1) the ascending uncrossed posterior trigeminal tract in the posterior tegmentum (Fig. 7.1), and (2) the ascending crossed anterior trigeminal tract. The anterior and posterior trigeminal tracts (Fig. 7.1) terminate in the ventral posteromedial thalamic nucleus and the posterior thalamic region, while the trigeminoreticulothalamic pathway terminates in the intralaminar nuclei of the thalamus (Chap. 7).

The *solitariothalamic tract* is composed of second-order *taste fibers* which originate in the gustatory portion of the nucleus of the solitary tract (input from ns. VII, IX, and X). It is apparently a crossed tract which ascends in association with the medial lemniscus and terminates in the ventral posteromedial thalamic nucleus.

The auditory and vestibular pathways passing through the brainstem tegmentum are discussed in Chap. 13. Brainstem structures involved with auditory pathways include the dorsal and ventral cochlear nuclei, trapezoid body, superior olivary nucleus, lateral lemniscus, inferior colliculus, and brachium of the inferior colliculus. Those involved with the vestibular system include the inferior, superior, lateral, and medial vestibular nuclei; medial longitudinal fasciculus; and lateral vestibulospinal tract.

BRAINSTEM: RETICULAR FORMATION

The *tegmental reticular* formation (Fig. 19.1) is an intricate neural network composed of reticular nuclei, ascending reticular pathways, descending reticular pathways, and local reflex arcs of cranial nerves. The ascending and descending intrinsic pathway interconnecting various levels of the brainstem reticular formation is the central tegmental tract (reticuloreticular fibers). The neurons of the reticular nuclei are anatomically oriented within the complex matrix of the tegmentum in a definite pattern: (1) The cell body and extensive dendritic arborization of each reticular neuron are oriented in the transverse plane (perpendicular to the long axis of the brainstem); (2) its axon generally bifurcates into a long ascending branch and a long descend-ing branch extending parallel to the long axis of the brainstem; each branch has many arborizing collaterals. The connectivity of a neuron within this tegmentum is rich and extensive; each neuron may receive synaptic input from over 4,000 other neurons (convergence) and, in turn, may have synaptic connections with over 25,000 other neurons (divergence). The reticular formation is the anatomic substrate for the physiologically defined reticular system (Chap. 19).

In general, the lateral third of the reticular formation, called the *sensory zone,* receives input from a variety of sources, whereas the medial two-thirds, called the *motor zone,* projects efferent output (Fig. 19.1). The input to the sensory zone is derived from (1) the spinal cord via the spinoreticular tracts and collateral branches of the spinothalamic and spinotectal tracts, (2) the cranial nerves, especially the trigeminal nerve, (3) the cerebrum via cortico-reticular, corticobulbar, and hypothalamotegmental pathways, and (4) the cerebellum via cerebelloreticular fibers. The output from the motor zone projects rostrally to the hypothalamus and thalamic intralaminar nuclei, caudally to the spinal cord via rubrospinal and reticulospinal tracts, and posteriorly to the cerebellum.

The main tract of the reticular formation of the brainstem tegmentum is the central tegmental tract. This tract is integrated into (1) the ascending reticular activating system (Chap. 19), (2) the spinoreticulothalamic pain pathway (Chap. 6), and (3) the corticorubrospinal, corticoreticulospinal, corticobulbar, and corticoreticular pathways (Chap. 9).

ASCENDING MONOAMINE PATHWAYS OF THE CNS

Several pathways have been identified and described in chemical as well as anatomic terms. The neurons of these pathways contain one of the following monoamines: norepinephrine, 5-hydroxytryptamine (serotonin, 5-HT), and dopamine. These monoamines are present in the cell bodies, axons, and endings of these neurons. Hence, they are collectively called *monoamine (aminergic, monoaminergic) neuronal pathways.* Evidence indicates that these monoamines and their precursors and associated enzymes are synthesized in the cell bodies of neurons and distributed in monoamine vesicles via axo-plasmic flow to the nerve terminals. These putative neurotransmitters are also synthesized in axon terminals. Neurons with norepinephrine comprise the *noradrenergic pathways* (Fig. 11.6); those with serotonin, the *serotoniner-gic pathways* (Fig. 21.4); and those with dopamine, the *dopaminergic path-ways* (Fig. 21.4).

Brainstem nuclei With respect to the brainstem, the cell bodies of the *noradrenergic neurons* are localized in the tegmentum of the pons and medulla (apparently they are absent in the midbrain tegmentum); those of the *serotoninergic neurons* are found in the raphe nuclei; and those of the *dopaminergic neurons* are restricted to the substantia nigra and to regions surrounding the interpeduncular nucleus of the midbrain.

Ascending Noradrenergic (NA) Pathway (Fig. 11.6)

Ascending NA fibers originate from cells of the brainstem reticular nuclei located (1) in the ventrolateral medulla, (2) in the lower pons dorsal and lateral to the superior olivary nuclei, and (3) in the upper pons ventral to the superior cerebellar peduncle. These fibers ascend as *the ventral NA pathways*

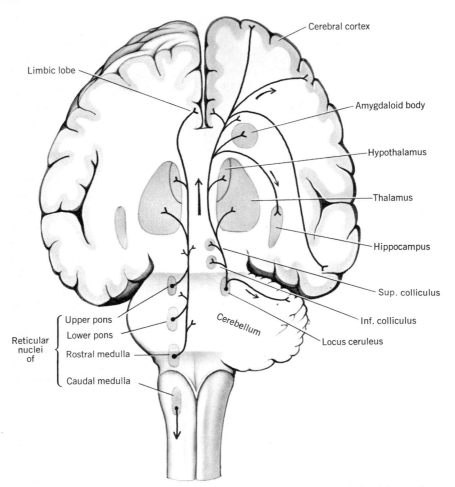

Figure 11.6 Noradrenergic pathways. The ascending pathway on the left originates from the medullary and pontine reticular nuclei and terminates in the cerebrum. The descending pathway on the left originates from medullary reticular nuclei and terminates in the spinal cord. The projections from the locus ceruleus on the right course (1) via the lateral pathway to the cerebellum and (2) via the ascending pathway to the midbrain and cerebrum.

within the medial and ventromedial brainstem reticular formation and medial forebrain bundle of the hypothalamus. The fibers of this pathway terminate as nerve endings in the lower brainstem, mesencephalon, and cerebrum. Some of the structures in which these fibers terminate include the dorsal vagal nucleus and nucleus solitarius of the medulla, some reticular nuclei and periaqueductal gray matter of the midbrain, hypothalamus, thalamus, and limbic lobe.

NA Pathways from the Locus Ceruleus (Fig. 11.6)

The *locus ceruleus* is composed largely of catecholamine-containing cell bodies, which contain norepinephrine. These cells give rise to the ascending pathway to the cerebrum called the *dorsal NA pathway,* and the *lateral pathway* to the cerebellum. This *dorsal pathway* is composed primarily of uncrossed fibers; a few of the fibers are crossed. These fibers from the locus ceruleus project directly as an ascending monosynaptic pathway (without interposed relay nuclei) to many regions of the brain, especially in the diencephalon and telencephalon. These include some brainstem nuclei such as the inferior and superior colliculi, thalamic nuclei, hypothalamus, amygdaloid body, septal area, hippocampus, and wide areas of the cerebral cortex. The terminals of NA fibers are present in all laminae of the cerebral cortex.

The fine fibers of the *lateral pathway* course through the ipsilateral superior cerebellar peduncle to all parts of the cerebellar cortex. Evidence indicates that these fibers exert inhibitory influences upon the distal segments of the dendritic tree of the Purkinje cells. It is likely that each cell body in the locus ceruleus has axonal branches, one of which terminates in the cerebellum and another in the cerebral cortex; in addition, collateral branches terminate in the midbrain colliculi, thalamus, and hypothalamus. These axons from one cell, which terminate monosynaptically in such diverse regions, may exert influences simultaneously in both the cerebral and cerebellar cortices. These projections influence and modify behavioral arousal, the electroencephalograph, the degree of "alertness" of cerebral cortex, and sleep.

Ascending Serotoninergic (5-HT) Pathway (Fig. 21.4)

The cell bodies of the raphe nuclei of the pons and lower midbrain (nucleus raphe pontis, superior central nucleus, and dorsal and ventral tegmental nuclei) have high concentrations of serotonin. Axons originating from these cell bodies form the ascending serotonin (5-HT) pathway. It ascends and terminates in the hypothalamus, amygdaloid body, septal nuclei, cingulate cortex, and neocortex.

These raphe nuclei are, in some way, related to various aspects of behavior and to the sleep-wake cycle. Total insomnia occurs when these raphe nuclei are destroyed or when the serotonin stores are depleted by the drug reserpine. In contrast, an increase in the brain serotonin level decreases the sensitivity to pain.

Dopaminergic (DA) Pathway (Fig. 21.4)

The cell bodies of the compact zone of the substantia nigra and of the region dorsal to the interpeduncular nucleus have high concentrations of dopamine

(DA). The axons originating in the compact zone ascend successively through the globus pallidum and internal capsule to the neostriatum (caudate nucleus and putamen). This *nigrostriatal DA system* is integrated in the basal ganglia circuits (Chap. 21). Some DA fibers from the substantia nigra terminate in the amygdaloid body. The fibers originating from the cells dorsal to the interpeduncular nucleus ascend within the medial forebrain bundle and terminate in the hypothalamus, amygdaloid body, and other portions of the limbic lobe. Some dopaminergic neurons project to the hypophysis. The reduction or depletion of DA in the nigrostriatal DA system is associated with paralysis agitans (Chap. 21).

DESCENDING PATHWAYS IN THE BASILAR PORTION

The corticospinal tract descends from widespread cortical areas successively through the rostral portion of the posterior limb of the internal capsule, middle portion of the crus cerebri, pons proper, and pyramids before decussating and entering the spinal cord. Some collateral branches do terminate in the brainstem reticular formation. Many fibers of the cortico-bulbar and corticoreticular tracts descend through the genu of the internal capsule, crus cerebri, and pons proper before terminating in neuronal pools stimulating motor nuclei of the cranial nerves (see Chap. 9) and nuclei of the brainstem reticular formation.

In addition, the descending pathway composed of the corticopontine tracts, pontine nuclei, and pontocerebellar tracts is located in the basilar portion of the midbrain and pons. The pathways and feedback circuits between the brainstem and the cerebellum are outlined in Chap. 15.

Chapter 12

Cranial Nerves

FUNCTIONAL COMPONENTS

The 12 cranial nerves are the peripheral nerves of the brain. Many have the same general functional components as are found in the spinal nerves: namely, general somatic afferent (GSA), general visceral afferent (GVA), general somatic efferent (GSE), and general visceral efferent (GVE) components. In addition, many cranial nerves have special components: namely, special somatic afferent (SSA), special visceral afferent (SVA), and special visceral (branchial) efferent (SVE) components. The terms defining the components are used as follows: *somatic* refers to head, body wall, and extremities; *visceral* to viscera; *afferent* to sensory (input); *efferent* to motor (output); *general* to wide areas of the head and body; *special* to the specialized functions of olfaction (smell), gustation (taste), sight, audition, equilibrium (vestibular system), and branchiomeric (gill arch) muscles. Some apparent inconsistencies in the use of these terms are prompted by their traditional use (e.g., branchiomeric voluntary muscles are called visceral because of their association with the visceral functions of eating and breathing).

101

CLASSIFICATION OF CRANIAL NERVES

On the basis of their functional components the cranial nerves may be placed into the following three categories. A few minor discrepancies are incorporated into this classification. The number of the nerve and its functional component are enclosed in parentheses.

Special Afferent Nerves

The olfactory nerve (n. I, SVA), optic nerve (n. II, SSA), and vestibulocochlear nerve (n. VIII, SSA) convey influences from special receptors. Taste fibers (SVA) are present in the visceral arch nerves, as noted below.

General Somatic Efferent Nerves

The oculomotor (n. III, GSE, GVE), trochlear (n. IV, GSE), abducent (n. VI, GSE), and hypoglossal (n. XII, GSE) nerves innervate the voluntary somatic (extraocular) muscles of the eye and tongue. Each of these nerves has fibers conveying proprioceptive (GSA) influences from the muscles to the brainstem. Nerve III has parasympathetic (GVE) fibers.

Visceral Arch (Branchiomeric) Nerves

The trigeminal (n. V, SVE, GSA), facial (n. VII, SVE, SVA, GVA), glossopharyngeal (n. IX, SVE, GVE, SVA, GVA), vagus (n. X, SVE, GVE, SVA, GVA), and spinal accessory (n. XI, SVE) nerves innervate the derivatives of the branchial (gill) arches and some additional structures. The first (jaw) arch is innervated by n. V, the second (hyoid) arch by n. VII, the third arch by n. IX, and the remaining arches by n. X. Note that ns. VII, IX, and X have the same functional components. The SVE fibers are lower motor neurons innervating the voluntary (striated) muscles of each arch. The GVE fibers are parasympathetic components of the autonomic nervous system. The SVA components are taste neurons. The ns. VII, IX, and X have a few GSA fiber components associated with cutaneous sensibility in the external auditory meatus, tympanic cavity, and a small area of external ear. For further information see the discussion of specific nerves below.

GANGLIA IN THE HEAD

The named ganglia in the head are of two types: (1) sensory ganglia containing the cell bodies of neurons of the first order (equivalent to the dorsal root ganglia), and (2) parasympathetic ganglia. The *sensory* ganglia including their associated cranial nerves and functional components are trigeminal (Gasserian, semilunar) ganglion (and mesencephalic nucleus of n. V, GSA); geniculate ganglion of n. VII (GVA, SVA, GSA); vestibular ganglion and spiral ganglia of n. VIII (SSA); superior (GSA) and inferior (SVA) ganglia of n. IX; and superior (GSA) and inferior (SVA) ganglia of n. X.

The *parasympathetic* ganglia (GVE), where preganglionic fibers synapse with postganglionic fibers, include the ciliary ganglion of n. III; pterygopalatine (sphenopalatine) and submandibular ganglia of n. VII; and the otic ganglion of n. IX.

CRANIAL NERVE NUCLEI WITHIN THE BRAINSTEM

The sensory nuclei of termination of the afferent fibers (Fig. 12.1) and the nuclei of origin of the motor fibers of the cranial nerves (Fig. 12.2) are organized in discontinuous nuclear "columns" within the brainstem. The olfactory nerve (n. I, SVA) and the optic nerve (n. II, SSA) are telencephalic and not brainstem cranial nerves.

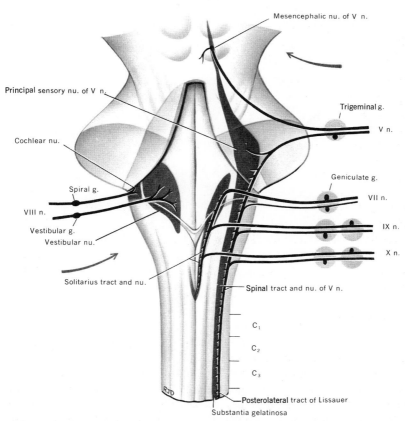

Figure 12.1 Location of the afferent (sensory) cranial nerve nuclei within the brainstem. These nuclei are organized into three nuclear columns. The superior and inferior ganglia of the ninth and tenth cranial nerves are not labeled; n. nerve.

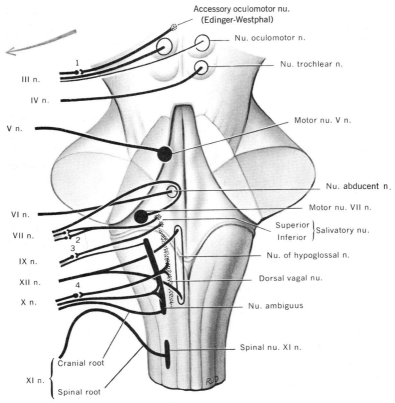

Figure 12.2 Location of the efferent (motor) cranial nerve nuclei within the brainstem. These nuclei are organized into three nuclear columns. Arabic numerals indicate parasympathetic ganglia: (1) ciliary ganglon, (2) pterygopalatine and submandibular ganglia, (3) otic ganglion, and (4) terminal ganglia.

Sensory Nuclei of Termination (Fig. 12.1)

The *special somatic afferent column* includes the vestibular and cochlear nuclei (n. VIII), which are located in the posterolateral tegmentum of the upper medulla and lower pons. The *general somatic afferent column* includes the mesencephalic nucleus of n. V (proprioception), located in the postero-medial midbrain tegmentum; the principal (chief or main) sensory nucleus of n. V (touch), located in lateral midpontine tegmentum; and the spinal trigeminal nucleus (pain and temperature), located in the lateral tegmentum of the lower pons, medulla, and the upper two cervical spinal levels (fibers from ns. V, VII, IX, and X have fibers terminating in these nuclei). The mesencephalic nucleus of n. V is actually composed of cell bodies of neurons of the first order; it is a displaced portion of the trigeminal ganglion. The *visceral afferent column* consists of the nucleus solitarius located in the midposterior tegmentum of the medulla; its components include taste (SVA) and other visceral influences (GVA) which are conveyed via fibers in three cranial nerves, ns. VII, IX, and X.

Motor Nuclei of Origin (Fig. 12.2)

The *general somatic efferent column* includes nuclei of the oculomotor nerve (midbrain), trochlear nerve (lower midbrain), abducent nerve (lower pons), and hypoglossal nerve (medulla). These nuclei, located in the posteromedial tegmentum, are composed of lower motor neurons innervating the voluntary muscles of the eye and tongue. The *general visceral efferent column* includes the accessory oculomotor nucleus of Edinger-Westphal (midbrain, n. III), the superior salivatory nucleus (posterior tegmentum of lower pons, n. VII), the inferior salivatory nucleus (posterior tegmentum of upper medulla, n. IX), and the dorsal motor nucleus of the vagus nerve (posterior tegmentum of medulla, n. X). These nuclei are composed of the cell bodies of preganglionic parasympathetic neurons of the autonomic nervous system. The salivatory nuclei are identifiable only by physiologic effects. The *special visceral (branchial) efferent column* includes the motor nucleus of the fifth nerve (midpons, n. V), motor nucleus of the seventh nerve (lower pons, n. VII), and nucleus ambiguus (medulla, ns. IX, X, and XI). These nuclei of the lower motor neurons to the branchiomeric muscles are located in the middle of the tegmentum.

SOME FUNCTIONAL AND CLINICAL CONSIDERATIONS OF THE CRANIAL NERVES

Olfactory (n. I)

The olfactory nerve is composed of bipolar SVA neurons of the olfactory mucosa which act as both receptors and neurons of the first order. Each neuron is an olfactory chemoceptor, transducer of a stimulus, and the transmitter of nerve impulses of the olfactory bulb. The total inability to smell is called *anosmia.*

Optic (n. II)

The bipolar cells of the retina are the SSA first-order neurons of the visual pathway. The optic nerve is actually a tract composed of axons of the ganglion cells of the retina (see Chap. 16).

Oculomotor (n. III), Trochlear (n. IV), and Abducent (n. VI)

These cranial nerves have lower motor neurons (GSE) which innervate the extraocular voluntary muscles and the levator palpebrae muscle (eyelid). The integrated actions of these nerves are responsible for the conjugate movements of the eye. Each nerve has proprioceptive (GSA) fibers, which may

Table 12.1 Cranial Nerves and Their Functional Components

Name	Components	Functions (major)
I. Olfactory nerve	Special visceral afferent	Smell
II. Optic nerve	Special somatic afferent	Vision
III. Oculomotor nerve*	General somatic efferent	Movements of eyes
	General visceral efferent (parasympathetic)	Pupillary constriction and accommodation
IV. Trochlear nerve*	General somatic efferent	Movements of eyes
V. Trigeminal nerve	Special visceral efferent	Muscles of mastication and eardrum tension
	General somatic afferent	General sensations from anterior half of head including face, nose, mouth, and meninges
VI. Abducent nerve*	General somatic efferent	Movements of eyes
VII. Facial nerve†	Special visceral efferent	Muscles of facial expression and tension on ear bones
	General visceral efferent (parasympathetic)	Lacrimation and salivation
	Special visceral afferent	Taste
	General visceral afferent	Visceral sensory
VIII. Vestibulocochlear nerve	Special somatic afferent	Hearing and equilibrium reception
IX. Glossopharyngeal nerve†	Special visceral efferent	Swallowing movements
	General visceral efferent (parasympathetic)	Salivation
	Special visceral afferent	Taste
	General visceral afferent	Visceral sensory
X. Vagus nerve† and cranial root of XI	Special visceral efferent	Swallowing movements and laryngeal control
	General visceral efferent (parasympathetic)	Parasympathetics to thoracic and abdominal viscera
	Special visceral afferent	Taste
	General visceral afferent	Visceral sensory
XI. Spinal accessory nerve (spinal root)	Special visceral efferent	Movements of shoulder and head
XII. Hypoglossal nerve*	General somatic efferent	Movements of tongue

* General somatic afferent—proprioception from the muscles of the eye (III, IV, VI) and tongue (XII).
† General somatic afferent—cutaneous sense from small portion of and just behind external ear.

have their cell bodies along the nerve, in the trigeminal ganglion, or in the mesencephalic nucleus of n. V. The third nerve has preganglionic parasympathetic (GVE) fibers synapsing with postganglionic neurons in the ciliary ganglion. They have a role in accommodation and pupillary constriction (see Chap. 16).

The precise role of these muscles in eye movements is complex, with the action of an individual muscle varying with the position of the eyeball within the orbit. The following account is schematic. Nerve III innervates the levator palpebrae, superior rectus, inferior rectus, medial rectus, and inferior oblique muscles. Nerve IV innervates the superior oblique muscle, and nerve VI innervates the lateral rectus muscle. The integrated activity of these muscles results in conjugate eye movements—horizontal, vertical, oblique, and converging—which cannot be voluntarily dissociated. The levator palpebrae muscle elevates the eyelid. The medial rectus is an *adductor* of the eye (pupil directed to nose), and the lateral rectus is an *abductor* (pupil directed to temple). These horizontal recti move the eyeball in the horizontal plane. In lateral gaze the medial rectus of one eye and the lateral rectus of the other eye contract synergistically. During convergence both medial recti contract. In contrast, the action of the muscles responsible for vertical movements—superior and inferior recti and superior and inferior oblique muscles—are influenced by the position of the eyeball in the orbit. The superior rectus elevates the eye (pupil up); the elevation increases with abduction. The inferior rectus depresses (pupil down); the depression increases with abduction. The superior oblique intorts (rotates the upper part medially) the abducted eye and depresses (moves pupil down) the adducted eye. Intorsion increases with greater abduction, and depression increases with greater adduction. The inferior oblique elevates the adducted eye and extorts the abducted eye.

The paralysis of one or more extraocular muscles results in *diplopia* (double vision) due to the faulty conjugate movements of the two eyes. Except for convergence, all normal eye movements are *conjugate* (conjugate movements); that is, the two eyes turn so that their visual axes remain parallel. A complete lesion of an oculomotor nerve produces the following: (1) *ptosis* or drooping of the eyelid and inability to elevate eyelid because of unopposed action of the orbicularis muscle which closes the eyelid (innervated by n. VII); (2) dilated pupil (*mydriasis*) and unresponsiveness of eye reflexes to light (pupillary constrictor and ciliary muscle paralysis from third nerve injury and the unopposed action of pupillary dilator muscle which is innervated by the intact sympathetic fibers); (3) pupils of unequal size (anisocoria); (4) external *strabismus* with the eye in abduction and unable to move inward, upward, and downward. This crossed horizontal diplopia is due to the unopposed action of the lateral rectus and the superior oblique muscles. The eye cannot be adducted or elevated.

A complete lesion of the trochlear nerve results in a vertical diplopia, head tilt, and limitation of ocular movement on looking down and in. Diplopia is maximal when the eyes are turned down; this makes it difficult for the subject to descend stairs. To align the eyes in order to minimize or eliminate the diplopia, the patient tilts his head to the shoulder of the side opposite the paralyzed muscle. Because the trochlear nerve decussates within the brainstem, the nucleus of the trochlear nerve is located on the side opposite to that of the trochlear nerve; hence a lesion of a nucleus of the trochlear nerve is expressed in the contralateral eye.

A complete lesion of the abducent nerve results in a horizontal diplopia with the ipsilateral eye adducted because of the unopposed action of the normal medial rectus muscle. Abduction is limited. The diplopia is maximal when the subject attempts to gaze to the side of the lesion (because the eye with the paralyzed lateral rectus muscle cannot be adequately abducted). It is minimal with gaze to the normal side because the visual axis of the normal eye can parallel that of the affected eye.

Trigeminal (n. V)

The trigeminal nerve is separated into three divisions: ophthalmic, maxillary, and mandibular. Each division supplies a distinct region; there is no overlap in the regions innervated by each of the three divisions (this contrasts with dermatomal overlap of spinal root distribution—see Chap. 5).

The sensory fibers enter at the midpons level as the sensory root (*portio major*), while the motor fibers emerge through the adjacent motor root (*portio minor*). The sensory input (GSA) is conveyed via first-order fibers (with cell bodies in the trigeminal ganglion) from the skin of the scalp anterior to the coronal plane through the ears (innervated regions include face, orbit, membranes of the nasal cavity, nasal sinuses and oral cavity, teeth, and most of the dura mater). These first-order neurons terminate in the principal sensory nucleus of n. V and in the spinal trigeminal nucleus (see also "Afferent Sensory Fibers," Chap. 11).

Some first-order neurons have their cell bodies in the mesencephalic nucleus of n. V; these proprioceptive neurons receiving input from the muscles of mastication are integrated with the motor nucleus of n. V into the two-neuron jaw reflex (compare with knee jerk reflex). The mesencephalic nucleus also receives proprioceptive input from the extraocular muscles. The lower motor neuron fibers from the motor nucleus of n. V (SVE) pass through the motor root and the mandibular division before innervating the jaw muscles of mastication (masseter, pterygoids, and temporalis muscles) and the tensor tympani and tensor palatini muscles. The jaw jerk can be evoked by tapping the chin of the slightly opened mouth.

The interruption of all trigeminal fibers unilaterally results in anesthesia and loss of general senses in the regions innervated by n. V and a lower motor neuron paralysis (weakness, fibrillations, loss of jaw jerk, and atrophy) of the jaw muscles. The sensory changes include loss in one nostril of the sensitivity of the nasal mucosa to ammonia and other volatile chemicals (smarting effect) and loss of corneal sensation on that side. The complete interruption of the sensory fibers from the cornea results in loss of the ipsilateral and contralateral (consensual) corneal reflex. The afferent limb of the corneal reflex (n. V) stimulates both efferent limbs through influences projected to both facial motor nuclei (n. VII), whose motor fibers innervate the orbicularis oculi muscles of both eyes. The loss of proprioceptive input may result in the relaxation of the ipsilateral muscles of facial expressions (innervated by n. VII). The loss of the jaw jerk results from the interruption of both the afferent and efferent limbs of the arc. Because of the action of the contracting pterygoid muscles on the normal side, the jaw, when protruded, will deviate and point to the paralyzed side. The patient may experience partial deafness to low-pitched sounds because of the paralysis of the tensor tympani muscle.

Sharp, agonizing pain localized over the distribution of one or more branches of the trigeminal nerve is known as *trigeminal neuralgia* or *tic douloureux*. This condition of unknown cause may be accompanied by muscle twitchings (tic) and disturbances in salivary secretion. The stimulation of a region, called a *trigger zone,* may initiate an attack.

The supranuclear influences upon the motor nucleus of n. V are outlined in Chap. 9. Because the motor nucleus of n. V is influenced by both crossed and uncrossed corticobulbar and corticoreticular pathways, unilateral supranuclear (upper motor neuron) lesions usually do not impair trigeminal motor activity.

Facial (n. VII)

The facial nerve consists of the facial nerve proper with its lower motor neurons (motor division, SVE) and the nervus intermedius with its sensory (GVA, SVA, GSA) components. All sensory neurons of the first order have their cell bodies in the geniculate ganglion. The GVA input from the viscera in the soft palate and tonsilar region and the SVA (taste) input from the anterior two-thirds of the tongue terminate in the nucleus solitarius. Taste fibers terminate in the rostral portion of nucleus solitarius (gustatory nucleus). Fibers from the motor nucleus of n. VII (SVE) take a hairpin course through the lower pons (they recurve as the internal genu around the nucleus of n. VI, Fig. 11.5E) before emerging into and passing through the cerebellopontine angle. These fibers innervate the muscles of facial expression, including the orbicularis oculi (closes eyelid and protects eye), buccinator (moves cheek), and stapedius (moves stapes bone) muscles. The parasympathetic preganglionic fibers from the superior salivatory nucleus have synaptic connections with postganglionic neurons in the pterygopalatine and submandibular ganglia; these fibers stimulate the lacrimal, nasal, oral, submaxillary, and sublingual glands and blood vessels.

A lesion interrupting the facial nerve (e.g., *Bell's palsy*) is primarily expressed as a lower motor neuron paralysis of the muscles of facial expression. The paresis of Bell's palsy may occur suddenly and be followed within a few months by a spontaneous recovery. On the ipsilateral side, the forehead is immobile, the corner of the mouth sags, the nasolabial folds of the face are flattened, facial lines are lost, and saliva may drip from the corner of the mouth. The patient is unable to whistle or puff the cheek because the buccinator muscle is paralyzed. When the patient is smiling, the normal muscles draw the contralateral corner of the mouth up while the paralyzed corner continues to sag. Corneal sensitivity remains (n. V), but the patient is unable to blink or close the eyelid (n. VII). To protect the cornea from damage (e.g., drying) therapeutic closure of eyelids or other measures are taken (e.g., patient wears an eye mask, or lids are closed by sutures). Lacrimation and salivation on the lesion side may be impaired. Taste will be lost on the ipsilateral anterior two-thirds of the tongue. An increased acuity to sounds (*hyperacusis*), especially to low tones, results from the paralysis of the stapedius muscle, which normally dampens the amplitude of the vibrations of the ear ossicles.

A unilateral supranuclear lesion of the upper motor neurons (corticobulbar and corticoreticular fibers) to the facial nucleus (see Chap. 14) results in a marked weakness of the muscles of expression of the face below the eye on the side contralateral to the lesion (Fig. 9.1). The frontalis muscle (wrinkles forehead) and the orbicularis oculi muscle (closes eyelid) are unaffected. The accepted explanation states that (1) bilateral upper motor neuron projections from the cerebral cortex influence the lower motor neurons innervating the frontalis muscle and orbicularis oculi, and (2) only unilateral, crossed upper motor neuron projections influence the lower motor neurons innervating the muscles of facial expression of the lower face. Hence the contralateral muscles are deprived of upper motor neuron influences.

In some patients with supranuclear lesions, the weak, lower facial muscles will remain paralyzed to volitional influences but will respond to emotional or mimetic influences (joke, distress). The influences that evoke this involuntary response are said to come from subcortical sources.

Note the distinction between a lower motor lesion and an upper motor lesion involving the muscles of facial expression (Fig. 9.1). In a lower motor paralysis the entire half of the face has marked weakness, whereas in an upper motor neuron only the lower half of the ipsilateral face has marked weakness.

Vestibulocochlear (n. VIII) (See Chap. 13)
Glossopharyngeal (n. IX)

The GVA input of n. IX from the palatine, tonsillar, and pharyngeal regions and from the carotid sinus (pressoreceptor, arterial pressure) and carotid body (chemoreceptor, CO_2 and O_2 concentration in blood) is conveyed via first-order fibers (cell bodies in superior ganglion) to the nucleus solitarius. The SVA input (taste) from the posterior third of the tongue is relayed via first-order neurons (cell bodies in inferior ganglion) to the nucleus solitarius. Some GSA afferents from the tympanic cavity and external auditory meatus terminate in the spinal trigeminal nucleus. The SVE lower motor neurons from the nucleus ambiguus innervate pharyngeal and palatine muscles (effect swallowing) and the stylopharyngeal muscle (elevates upper pharynx). The preganglionic parasympathetic (GVE) influences from the inferior salivatory nucleus are relayed via the otic ganglion to the parotid gland.

Interruption of all fibers of n. IX results in the following symptoms: (1) loss of sensation, including taste, in the posterior third of the tongue and adjacent area; (2) unilateral loss of gag (pharyngeal) and palatal, uvular, and carotid reflexes; and (3) difficulty in swallowing (*dysphagia*) and deviation of palate and uvula to the normal side (unopposed by paralyzed muscles). Glossopharyngeal neuralgia (similar to trigeminal neuralgia) may be triggered by chewing or swallowing.

Vagus (n. X)

The GVA input of n. X from the respiratory system (larynx, trachea, and lungs), cardiovascular system (carotid sinus and body, heart, various blood vessels), gastrointestinal tract (including pharynx and esophagus), and dura mater of the posterior fossa and the SVA (taste) input from the epiglottis are conveyed via first-order neurons (cell bodies in superior, GVA, and inferior, SVA, ganglia) to the nucleus solitarius. The general somatic afferents from the external auditory meatus terminate in the spinal trigeminal nucleus. The SVE lower motor neurons from the nucleus ambiguus innervate the voluntary muscles of the soft palate, pharynx, and intrinsic laryngeal muscles (some of these fibers from the nucleus ambiguus course via n. XI before joining the vagus nerve). The preganglionic parasympathetic influences (GVE) from the dorsal vagal nucleus are relayed via postganglionic neurons in terminal ganglia to the cardiovascular, respiratory, and gastrointestinal systems of the thorax and abdomen (see Chap. 17). Preganglionic parasympathetic neurons to the heart may arise from cells located close to the nucleus ambiguus.

A complete unilateral lesion of the vagus nerve results in the following symptoms: (1) The flaccid soft palate produces a voice with a twang; (2)

swallowing is difficult (*dysphagia*) because of the unilateral paralysis of pharyngeal constrictors; the pharynx is shifted slightly to the normally innervated side. A transient *tachycardia* (increased heartbeat) is a consequence of the interruption of some parasympathetic stimulation. (See "Accessory Nerve" below for reference to lesion of the recurrent laryngeal nerve.) Bilateral lesions of the vagus nerves may be rapidly fatal because of laryngeal paralyses of the adducted vocal folds.

Accessory (Spinal Accessory) (n. XI)

The accessory nerve consists of two roots, spinal and bulbar (cranial). The fibers of the spinal root originate from the anterior horn cells of cervical levels 1 through 5, emerge, and ascend on the side of the spinal cord (dorsal to the denticulate ligament) and medulla, and join the cranial root in the jugular foramen; the spinal root innervates the ipsilateral sternomastoid and the upper half of the trapezius muscles. The fibers of the cranial root originate from the nucleus ambiguus, course with n. XI a short distance before branching and joining n. X, and eventually form the recurrent laryngeal nerve which innervates the intrinsic laryngeal muscles.

The lower motor neuron paralysis of the spinal root fibers is indicated by a weakness in the ability to rotate the head so that the chin points to the side opposite the lesion (paralyzed sternomastoid muscle) and in a downward and outward rotation of the upper scapula (paralyzed upper trapezius muscle). After a unilateral lesion of the cranial root fibers (or recurrent laryngeal nerve), the ipsilateral vocal cord becomes fixed and partially adducted; the voice is hoarse (*dysphonia*) and reduced to a whisper.

Hypoglossal (n. XII)

The lower motor neuron fibers originate in the nucleus of the hypoglossal nerve and innervate the ipsilateral tongue musculature, including its intrinsic muscles and the genioglossus, styloglossus, and hypoglossus. Interruption of the fibers of n. XII produces an ipsilateral lower motor neuron paralysis of the tongue. The fibrillations of the early stages are followed by atrophy of muscles, which results in a wrinkled tongue surface on the side of the lesion. When protruded, the tongue deviates to the paralyzed side. The deviation is due to the unopposed contraction of the contralateral genioglossus, which pulls the base of the tongue forward.

Chapter 13

Auditory and Vestibular Systems

eliminate
except for p. 120 and
overlap with lecture

The exteroceptive auditory system concerned with hearing and the proprioceptive vestibular system concerned with the maintenance of equilibrium and the orientation of the body in space have their sensors located within the inner ears. The receptors—actually mechanoreceptors—are hair cells within specialized neuroepithelial structures of the membranous labyrinth, which is a closed tubular system filled with endolymph. The input from the auditory receptors in the spiral organ of Corti in the cochlea is conveyed via fibers of the cochlear nerve to the auditory pathways. The input from the vestibular receptors located in the macula of the utricle, the macula of the saccule, and the cristae ampullae of the three semicircular canals is conveyed via fibers of the vestibular nerve to the vestibular pathways. The cochlear nerve and the vestibular nerve are called the vestibulocochlear nerve or the eighth cranial nerve (n. VIII), which traverses the cerebellopontine angle before entering the upper medulla.

113

AUDITORY SYSTEM

Ear

Vibrations may be perceived as sounds. Although frequencies between 50 to 16,000 cycles per second can be detected as sound, the frequencies perceived with optimum acuity by most subjects range between 2,000 and 5,000 cycles per second. Airborne vibrations pass through the *external auditory meatus* of the external ear, and they set the *tympanic membrane* (*eardrum*) vibrating. The membrane and the ear *ossicles* (*malleus, incus,* and *stapes*) within the middle ear constitute a most efficient impedance-matching apparatus for conveying the airborne vibrations at the oval window to the perilymphatic fluid of the cochlea of the inner ear. Solid-borne vibrations (bone conduction) may bypass the ear ossicles and reach the perilymphatic fluid directly. The vibratory pressure waves of the perilymphatic fluid are transmitted (1) up the scala vestibuli and down the scala tympani through the $2\frac{1}{2}$ turns of the cochlea, (2) to the vestibular (Reissner's) membrane, basilar membrane, and endolymphatic fluid of the cochlear duct, and (3) to the spiral organ of Corti and the tectorial membrane. The distal tips of the cilia of the hair cells of the spiral organ of Corti are embedded in the rigid keratinlike tectorial membrane (Fig. 13.1). The 140 or so cilia on each of the approximately 30,000 hair cells of the spiral organ of Corti vibrate with a shearing motion produced by the differential vibration of the spiral organ of Corti and the tectorial membrane. The hair cells are polarized, with stimulation occurring when the cilia are bent in one direction (axis of sensitivity). The highest pitches are monitored at the base of the coil of the spiral organ, the lowest tones at the apex, and the intermediate pitches in an organized pattern between the highest and the lowest (*tonotopic* organization). The loudness perceived is related to the amplitude of the vibration of the spiral organ of Corti. The effects of the stimulation are transmitted at the base of the hair cells to the nerve endings of the bipolar neurons of the spiral ganglion of the cochlear nerve.

Ascending Pathways (Fig. 13.2)

Each of the approximately 30,000 nerve fibers of the cochlear nerve has (1) distal branches terminating as synaptic connections with from a few to many hair cells of the spiral organ of Corti, and (2) proximal branches synapsing with many neurons in both the dorsal and ventral cochlear nuclei located on the posterolateral surface of the upper medulla. Most of the fibers from the cell bodies in the tonotopically organized cochlear nuclei decussate to the opposite side in the lower pons and ascend as the lateral lemniscus. The fibers from the ventral cochlear nucleus cross as the trapezoid body in the anterior pontine tegmentum, and those from the dorsal cochlear nuclei as the posterior and intermediate acoustic striae in the pos-

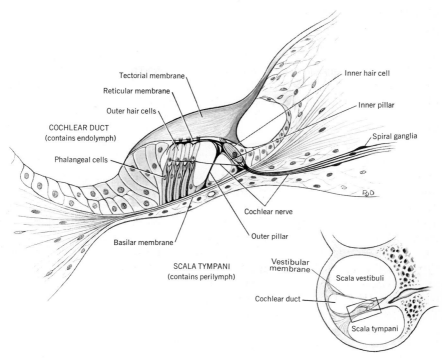

Figure 13.1 The spiral organ of Corti.

terior pontine tegmentum. Some fibers from the cochlear nuclei ascend as uncrossed fibers in the ipsilateral *lateral lemniscus.*

Intercalated within the ascending auditory pathways to the auditory cortex are several nuclei; these include the superior olivary nuclei, nucleus of trapezoid body, nucleus of lateral lemniscus, inferior colliculus, and medial geniculate body. Commissural fibers interconnect the bilateral inferior colliculi, which are tonotopically organized. The portion of the lateral lemniscus between the inferior colliculus and the medial geniculate body is called the *brachium* of the inferior colliculus. The fibers (auditory radiation) from the neurons of the medial geniculate body ascend through the posterior limb of the internal capsule (sublenticular portion) and terminate in the transverse gyri of Heschl (areas 41 and 42) of the temporal lobe. The medial geniculate body and the transverse gyri of Heschl may not exhibit sharp tonotopic localization.

Descending Pathways

Projecting from the cerebral cortex and the other nuclei of the auditory pathways are descending fibers within the auditory pathways (Fig. 13.2);

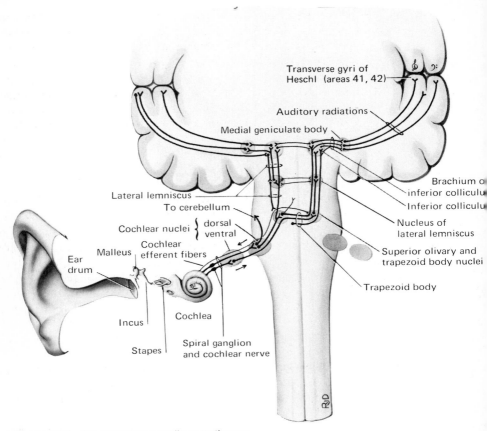

Figure 13.2 Diagram of the auditory pathways.

these fibers conveying descending influences have a role in processing ascending influences (they enhance signals and suppress noise). The nerve fibers from the superior olivary nuclei are integrated into a feedback system which courses as crossed and uncrossed projections—called the *olivocochlear* or *cochlear efferent bundle*—via the vestibulocochlear nerve, before terminating at the base of the hair cells of the spiral organ of Corti. The inhibitory influences conveyed via the olivocochlear fibers act to suppress the activity of the afferent fibers of the cochlear nerve.

Functional and Clinical Considerations

Complete damage of the cochlea or the cochlear nerve results in complete deafness in one ear. Usually complete deafness in one ear denotes nerve involvement (nerve deafness). Unilateral lesions of the ascending auditory pathways may be accompanied by a bilateral diminution of hearing acuity, which is more marked on the contralateral side. This is related to the fact that the ascending auditory pathways are composed mainly of crossed fibers. Lesions of the central auditory pathway do not lead to deafness unless they are bilateral.

An irritative lesion of the spiral organ of Corti or the cochlear nerve may result in *tinnitus*—the subjective hearing of hissing, roaring, buzzing, and humming sounds. This may occur in acoustic neuromas of n. VIII in the cerebellopontine angle. Tinnitus may be followed by nerve deafness as the irritative lesion expands and all cochlear nerve fibers are interrupted. The fibers of the vestibulocochlear nerve are sensitive to such drugs as streptomycin and aspirin; one of their toxic effects may be tinnitus.

Damage to the eardrum and the ossicles of the middle ear is usually followed by a partial deafness. This middle-ear deafness (conduction deafness in otosclerosis) is accompanied by a partial loss in the perception of low-pitched sounds and a mild loss in the entire auditory range.

The auditory pathways are reflexly integrated with the cranial nerves innervating the stapedius muscle (n. VII) and the tensor tympani (n. V). Immediately after stimulation by sounds of high intensity, these two muscles contract reflexly and exert tension on these ear ossicles; this action protects the spiral organ of Corti from damage by excessive stimulation. Paralysis of these muscles results in *hyperacusis*—the increased acuity of hearing and hypersensitivity to low tones.

The medial geniculate bodies are considered to be significant in the role of the recognition of pitch and sound intensity. Following the bilateral destruction of the auditory cortex, these qualities can still be appreciated.

VESTIBULAR SYSTEM

The receptor end organs in each ear of the vestibular system include the three cristae ampullares (one crista located in the ampulla of each semicircular canal) and the maculae of the utricle and of the saccule. The three semicircular canals, oriented at right angles to one another, represent the three dimensions in space. The 75 to 100 *stereocilia* (*hairs*) and one *kinocilium* of each hair cell of the many in each crista or macula are embedded in a gelatinous matrix which abuts against the roof of the ampulla; each cell is polarized with the kinocilium located to one side of all stereocilia (Fig. 13.3). The response of the hair cell is facilitatory when the hair bends in the direction of the kinocilium and inhibitory if bent in the opposite direction. All hair cells in each crista are polarized in the same direction (axis of sensitivity—Fig. 13.3). The cristae respond to angular movements of the head (not movement in a straight line); the movement of the endolymphatic fluid within the semicircular canals as the head turns and rotates results in the

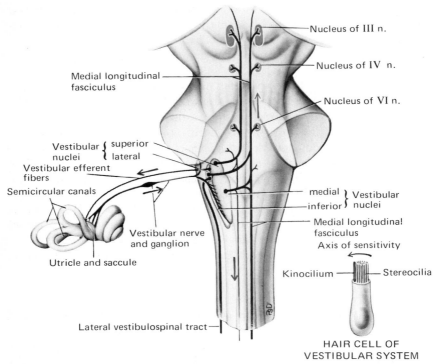

Figure 13.3 Diagram of pathways composing the vestibular nerve, vestibular nuclei, medial longitudinal fasciculus, and lateral vestibulospinal tract. The connections of the vestibular system with the vestibulocerebellum are illustrated in Fig. 15.4. The axis of sensitivity of a vestibular hair cell is in the direction of the kinocilium.

bending of the gelatinous matrix and the cilia and the triggering of facilitatory or inhibitory effects. The macula of the saccule is oriented with its long axis essentially in a vertical plane, and the macula of the utricle is basically oriented with its long axis in the horizontal plane. The stereocilia and kinocilium of each hair cell are embedded in a gelatinous matrix with calcareous otolith crystals; all hair cells are polarized. The *saccular macula* responds to vertically directed acceleratory and deceleratory linear displacements and gravity (e.g., movements up and down in an elevator). The *utricular macula* responds to horizontally directed forces and gravity. The saccule is said, by some investigators, to be a sensor for the reception of vibratory stimuli.

The role of the vestibular receptors in the orientation of the head and body in space is expressed through muscular activities in the coordination of eye reflexes, head position, and body movements. These specialized proprioceptors tend to (1) reinforce the tonic activity of muscles while the subject is in a stationary position (e.g., maintain balance while he is standing in a moving vehicle) and (2) trigger muscular reflexes in response to changes in the position of the head, body, and extremities (e.g., sustain balance while walking a tightrope).

Input to the Vestibular Nuclei (Fig. 13.3)

The bipolar neurons of the vestibular nerve (cell bodies in the vestibular ganglion) terminate distally by synapsing with the hair cells of the vestibular receptors (maculae and cristae ampullares). Most of their centrally directed axons terminate within the brainstem in precise synaptic patterns within each of the four vestibular nuclei (superior, lateral, medial, and inferior), and, after coursing through the juxtarestiform body, other fibers terminate directly in the ipsilateral cerebellar cortex (primarily in the flocculonodular lobe). Fibers from the vestibulocerebellum and the fastigial nuclei of the cerebellum project to the vestibular nuclei (Chap. 15). In summary, the vestibular nuclei receive their main input from both the vestibular receptors and the cerebellum. In addition, the vestibular nuclei have reciprocal connections with the vestibulocerebellum and nuclei fastigii of the cerebellum (see Chap. 15).

Output from the Vestibular Nuclei

The influences from the vestibular nuclei are projected (1) to the spinal cord via the (lateral) vestibulospinal tract and medial vestibulospinal tract (Chap. 5), (2) to the cerebellum via fibers in the juxtarestiform body (Chap. 15), (3) to the brainstem primarily via the medial longitudinal fasciculus (vestibulo-mesencephalic fibers), and (4) via relays in the medial geniculate body to the temporal lobe cortex.

The *vestibulospinal tract* from the lateral vestibular nucleus is an ipsilateral, somatotopically organized bundle of fibers terminating in laminae VII and VIII at all levels of the spinal cord (see Fig. 9.2); it conveys facilitatory influences to extensor muscle tone and spinal reflexes. The *medial vestibulospinal tract* from the medial vestibular nucleus is primarily a crossed bundle of fibers descending in the medial longitudinal fasciculus before terminating in lamina VIII in the cervical and upper thoracic levels; it conveys inhibitory influences to extensor muscle tone.

Stimuli originating in the vestibular receptors may produce conjugate movements of the eyes (e.g., such coupled deviation of the two eyes as in nystagmus—see below). These vestibular influences are conveyed via the *medial longitudinal fasciculus (MLF)* to interneurons which interact with the lower motor neurons of ns. III, IV, and VI innervating the extraocular muscles. The fibers from the superior vestibular nucleus ascend in the ipsilateral MLF; those from the medial vestibular nucleus ascend in both the ipsilateral and contralateral MLFs; those from the lateral vestibular nucleus ascend in the contralateral MLF; and a few fibers from the inferior vestibular nucleus ascend in the MLF.

Vestibular influences are presumed to be projected rostrally via relays in the medial geniculate body to a vestibular cortical area near the auditory cortex. This pathway may be related to objective sensations (e.g., dizziness) associated with the vestibular system.

Vestibular Efferent Fibers

Central influences are conveyed via efferent fibers from the vestibular nuclei which pass through the vestibular nerve and terminate on the hair cells of the vestibular end organs (see *cochlear efferent bundle* in "Descending Pathways" above). These vestibular efferent fibers probably exert inhibitory effects which ameliorate influences that might result in motion sickness and nystagmus.

Functional and Clinical Considerations

Nystagmus is the rapid rhythmic oscillatory involuntary movement of one or both eyes in which a rapid movement in one direction is followed by a slow movement in the opposite direction. The nystagmus is usually conjugate in the horizontal plane but can also be in the vertical, oblique, or rotary planes. The direction of the nystagmus is defined by the direction of the fast component. The movement of the endolymph in relation to the cristae ampullae of the horizontal semicircular canals is the basis of the horizontal nystagmus—subjectively sensed as a whirling sensation after being rapidly spun in one direction for about 10 to 12 turns and suddenly brought to a halt. The direction of the nystagmus after stopping is in the opposite direction to the direction of the spin—that is, the fast component of the nystagmus is, after stopping, opposite to the direction of the original spin. The feeling of a whirling sensation is called *vertigo*. Any set of semicircular canals can be stimulated by holding the head in the proper plane and rotating the subject in a Barany chair; after the spinning of the chair is stopped, the nature of the nystagmus can be used to determine the functional status of the various canals. The semicircular canals can be tested calorically by the introduction of cold (or warm) water in the external auditory meatus—this sets up convection currents in the endolymph. Normally the nystagmus is to the same side after warm water is used (and to the opposite side after cold water is used).

Dizziness, feeling of lightheadedness, headache, nausea, and vomiting are symptoms associated with *motion sickness* (*seasickness* and *airsickness*). They are due primarily to the overstimulation of the maculae of the saccule and utricle. Deaf mutes, who lack receptors in the membranous labyrinths, do not experience motion sickness. Drugs such as Dramamine lower the threshold of vestibular stimulation and, thereby, ameliorate the symptoms of motion sickness.

Chapter 14

Lesions of the Brainstem

not responsible for

GENERAL CONSIDERATIONS

In general, the tracts passing through and within the brainstem are oriented in a longitudinal plane parallel to the long axis of the brainstem (e.g., spinal trigeminal tract, medial lemniscus, and pyramidal tract), while the cranial nerves course through a coronal plane perpendicular to the long axis (e.g., facial nerve). These orientations should be kept in mind in the following account.

The effect of any lesion will depend on the anatomic features of the nerve tracts which are interrupted and on the total innervation of the areas of the body and head affected by the lesion. Lesions of the following pathways within the brainstem result in signs on the opposite side of the body and occiput because these are *crossed* tracts: spinothalamic (decussates in spinal cord), medial lemniscus (decussates in lower medulla), and corticospinal (decussates in lower medulla). In their courses through the brainstem, (1) the spinothalamic tract is located in the lateral tegmentum, (2) the medial lemniscus shifts as it ascends from its location in the anteromedial tegmentum in the medulla to the posterolateral tegmentum in the midbrain before terminating in the ventral posterior lateral thalamic nucleus, and (3) the corticospinal tract descends through the medial portion of the brainstem.

A unilateral lesion of the auditory pathway (lateral lemniscus and brachium of the inferior colliculus) results in the diminution of hearing in both ears, but the diminution is greater in the contralateral ear. This occurs because each auditory pathway conveys influences from both ears, but *mainly* from the ear contralateral to the pathway.

A unilateral lesion of the anterior trigeminothalamic tract is accompanied by loss of pain and temperature on the forehead, face, nasal cavity, and oral cavity on the opposite side. This occurs because the lesion is *above* the level where the fibers of this tract decussate in the medulla.

Because the cranial nerves are oriented at right angles to the long axis of the brainstem, they can be helpful in *localizing* the level of a lesion. Nerves III (midbrain), VI (pons-medulla junction), and XII (medulla) emerge on the anterior aspect of the brainstem in close proximity to the descending corticospinal tract. Injury to one of these nerves and the corticospinal tract results in an *alternating hemiplegia*—lesion to the nerve is accompanied by a lower motor neuron paralysis on *same side* and lesion to the corticospinal tract by an upper motor neuron paralysis on the *opposite side* of body (lesion of corticospinal tract rostral to the level of its decussation).

The branchiomeric nerves (ns. V, VII, IX, X, and XI) pass close to the spinothalamic tract before emerging on the lateral side of the brainstem. Injury to one of these nerves and the spinothalamic tract results in (1) sensory loss of the region and a lower motor neuron paralysis of the muscles innervated by that nerve, and (2) loss of pain and temperature on the opposite side of the body and back of the head due to the interruption of the decussated fibers of the spinothalamic tract.

Blood Supply of the Brainstem

The sequence of vertebral arteries, basilar artery, and posterior cerebral arteries forms the main trunk system supplying arterial blood to the medulla, pons, midbrain, cerebellum, and posterior medial cerebrum (Fig. 3.1). The paired vertebral arteries ascend along the anterolateral aspect of the medulla and join at the pons-medulla junction to form the single medial basilar artery, which ascends and then divides in the midbrain region into the paired posterior cerebral arteries. Branches of these arteries supply the brainstem in patterns which may be conceptually summarized as follows: in a general way, the paramedian branches are distributed to a medial zone on either side of the midsagittal plane, the short circumferential branches to an anterolateral zone, and the long circumferential branches to a posterolateral zone and to the cerebellum (Fig. 14.1).

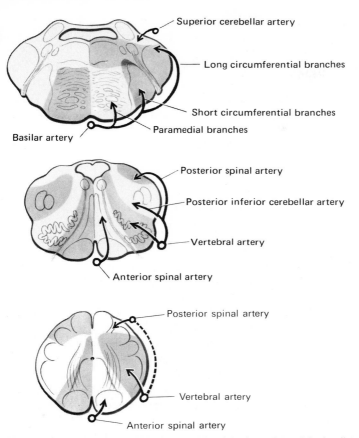

Figure 14.1 The patterns of arterial supply of the branches of the basilar artery within the pons (upper), midmedulla (middle), and caudal medulla (lower). Refer to Fig. 3.1.

MEDIAL ZONE OF THE MEDULLA (Fig. 14.2A)

The occlusion of an anterior spinal artery and its paramedian branches to the medial zone of the medulla may be the cause of a lesion which involves the hypoglossal nerve (n. XII), corticospinal tract of the pyramid, and medial lemniscus. This *alternating hemiplegia* combines a lower motor neuron paralysis of the tongue on the ipsilateral side (n. XII) with an upper motor neuron paralysis and a loss of discriminatory general senses (medial lemniscus) on the contralateral side of the body. During the first few weeks after the lesion, the ipsilateral half of the tongue will fibrillate (denervation sensitivity); later the muscles atrophy, and that side of the tongue appears wrinkled. When protruded, the tongue deviates to the paralyzed side; this is

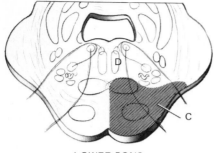

LOWER PONS

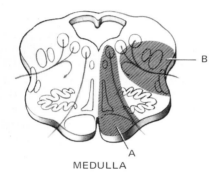

MEDULLA

Figure 14.2 Sites of lesions in the lower brainstem as described in the text. In the medulla, the lesions are located in the medial zone (A) and in the postero-lateral medulla (B). In the lower pons, the lesions are located in the medial and basal portion (C) and in the medial longitudinal fasciculus (D).

due primarily to the unopposed action of the contralateral genioglossus muscle. The contralateral side of the body exhibits the signs of an upper motor neuron paralysis (corticospinal tract) and loss of position, muscle, and joint sense, impaired tactile discrimination, and loss of vibratory sense (medial lemniscus), because the lesion interrupts these tracts above the level of their decussation.

POSTEROLATERAL MEDULLA (Fig. 14.2B)

The failure of the posterior inferior cerebellar artery (a long circumferential artery) may be the cause of a lesion resulting in the syndrome of the posterior inferior cerebellar artery (*lateral medullary syndrome*). Damage to the following structures will produce the symptoms: spinothalamic tract, spinal trigeminal tract and nucleus, fibers and possibly nuclei associated with the glossopharyngeal, vagal, and spinal portions of accessory nerves (including the nucleus ambiguus, dorsal vagal nucleus, and tractus and nucleus solitarius), part of the reticular formation, portions of the vestibular nuclei, and some fibers of the inferior cerebellar peduncle. The symptoms include (1) loss of pain (*analgesia*) and temperature (*thermoanesthesia*) on the opposite side of the body including the back of the head (crossed spinothalamic tract); (2) loss of pain and temperature on same side of face and nasal and oral cavities in all three trigeminal divisions (uncrossed spinal trigeminal tract and nucleus); (3) difficulty in swallowing (*dysphagia*) and a voice that is hoarse and weak (damage of nucleus ambiguus produces a lower motor neuron paralysis of the ipsilateral pharyngeal and laryngeal muscles—bulbar palsy; the normal palatal muscles will deviate the uvula to the normal side); (4) loss of gag reflex on the ipsilateral side and absence of sensation on ipsilateral side of fauces (glossopharyngeal nerve).

A bulbar palsy results following degeneration of motor neurons of the brainstem: A transient tachycardia (increase in heartbeat) may result from sudden withdrawal of some parasympathetic innervation; compensatory mechanisms including influences from the contralateral vagus nerve restore normal heartbeat. The absence of visceral afferent stimulation from some visceral receptors (e.g., carotid body and carotid sinus) to the solitary nucleus is compensated for by the input from similar receptors to the normal contralateral side. The interruption of fibers passing through the inferior cerebellar peduncle results in some signs of cerebellar malfunction on the ipsilateral side of the body—including hypotonia, asynergia, and poorly coordinated voluntary movements (Chap. 15). Irritation of the vestibular nuclei may be expressed by nystagmus or a deviation of eyes to the ipsilateral side. Horner's syndrome on the same side may occur if many descending fibers of the autonomic nervous system to the thoracic sympathetic outflow are damaged. The tactile and discriminative general senses from the face are normal because the principal sensory nucleus of n. V and its ascending pathways are above the lesion.

REGION OF THE CEREBELLOPONTINE ANGLE (CEREBELLOPONTINE ANGLE SYNDROME)

The slowly growing acoustic neuroma, which originates from neurolemmal cells of the vestibular nerve in the vicinity of the internal auditory foramen, may extend into the *cerebellopontine angle*—the junctional region of the cerebellum, pons, and medulla near the emergence of cranial nerves VII and VIII. In the early stages, symptoms are referable to the VIIIth cranial nerve; they include (1) tinnitus followed by progressive deafness on the lesion side, and (2) abnormal labyrinthine responses such as tilting and rotation of the head with the chin pointing to the lesion side. Later the tumor exerts pressure upon the brainstem and damages the fibers of the inferior and middle cerebellar peduncles, spinothalamic tract, spinal trigeminal tract, and facial nerve. The cerebellar signs which result from the involvement of the cerebellar peduncles include coarse intention tremor, dysmetria, moderate ataxic gait, adiadochokinesis, and others on the lesion side (Chap. 15). The loss of pain and temperature on the ipsilateral side of the face, oral cavity, and nasal cavity and on the contralateral side of the body are a consequence of damage to the spinal trigeminal tract and the spinothalamic tract, respectively; this combination of ipsilateral and contralateral sensory loss is called *alternating hemianesthesia.* Injury to the facial nerve may result in a lower motor paralysis of the muscles of facial expression (Bell's palsy), hyperacusis, and loss of taste on the anterior two-thirds of the tongue ipsilaterally (Chap. 12).

MEDIAL AND BASAL PORTION
OF THE CAUDAL PONS

The occlusion of paramedian and short circumferential branches of the basilar artery may result in damage to the following structures within the confines of the lesion: abducent nerve (n. VI), facial nerve (n. VII), pyramidal tract, medial lemniscus, and medial longitudinal fasciculus. The interruption of the fibers of n. VI (lower motor neurons) and the pyramidal tract (upper motor neurons) results in an *alternating abducent hemiplegia.* (Remember that in an alternating hemiplegia, the lower motor neuron paralysis is expressed on one side and the upper motor neuron paralysis is expressed on the opposite side.) The transection of n. VI produces a horizontal diplopia (double vision) due to the paralysis of the lateral rectus muscle (an abductor), as a consequence of which the image of an object falls upon noncorresponding portions of the two retinas and is seen as two objects. The diplopia is maximal when the patient attempts to gaze to the lesion side. When the ipsilateral lateral rectus muscle, which is innervated by n. VI, is paralyzed, the subject's ability to abduct the eye (pupil directed to temple) is impaired. The signs occurring from damage to the corticospinal fibers, VIIth nerve, and medial lemniscus are discussed above and the medial longitudinal fasciculus below.

MEDIAL LONGITUDINAL FASCICULUS (Fig. 14.2D)

A unilateral lesion of the medial longitudinal fasciculus (MLF) rostral to the nucleus of the abducent nerve results in a disturbance of conjugate horizontal eye movements (abduction and adduction) called *internuclear ophthalmoplegia.* Such lesions may occur in multiple sclerosis. This *lateral-gaze paralysis* is characterized by an impaired adduction of the ipsilateral eye and nystagmus of the abducting contralateral eye on gaze to the side opposite the lesion. This paralysis is due to the damage of the fibers which interconnect and integrate, during lateral gaze, the contraction of the contralateral lateral rectus muscle (abductor innervated by n. VI) and the ipsilateral medial rectus muscle (adductor innervated by n. III). In essence, the lateral rectus muscle of one eye (abducent) is yoked to the medial rectus muscle (oculomotor) in order to produce a coordinated lateral gaze. The weakness of the ipsilateral medial rectus muscle is due to the absence of influences derived from the ascending fibers in the MLF. These fibers cross at the level of the abducent nucleus. The horizontal diplopia is most marked during maximal lateral gaze to the contralateral side because the paralyzed ipsilateral medial rectus muscle is unable to adduct the eye. Lateral gaze to the side of the lesion is essentially conjugate because the pathways integrating the contractions of the ipsilateral lateral rectus muscle and the contralateral medial rectus muscle are intact.

LATERAL HALF OF THE MIDPONS

The structures within the region of the lesion (Fig. 14.3A) include the trigeminal nerve, spinothalamic tract, lateral lemniscus, and the middle cerebellar peduncle. Damage to the trigeminal nerve (n. V) results in (1) the absence of all general senses (anesthesia) on the ipsilateral side of the face, forehead, nasal cavity, and oral cavity—including absence of corneal sensation and corneal reflex—and (2) a lower motor neuron paralysis of the muscles of mastication with the chin deviating to the lesion side when the mouth is opened. If the lesion is extensive enough to include the corticospinal tract, the combination of the pyramidal tract and n. V produces an *alternating trigeminal hemiplegia.* The lesion of the lateral lemniscus may be followed by a diminution of audition, which is more marked on the opposite side (the lateral lemniscus is composed of fibers conveying some auditory influences from the same side but mainly from the opposite side). Interruption of pontocerebellar fibers may be expressed with some cerebellar signs on the same side (Chap. 15) including hypotonia, coarse intention tremor, and tendency to fall to the side of the lesion.

BASAL REGION OF THE MIDBRAIN

The occlusion of paramedian branches and short circumferential branches of the basilar and posterior cerebral arteries may produce a *Weber's syndrome* (Fig. 14.3B) which is a consequence of damage to the oculomotor nerve (n. III), the corticospinal tract, and a variable number of corticobulbar and corticoreticular fibers. The interruption of all the fibers in the oculomotor nerve results in signs restricted to the ipsilateral eye including drooping of eyelid (*ptosis,* or inability to raise eyelid because of paralysis of levator palpebral muscle), diplopia, external *strabismus* (squint) due to unopposed contraction of the lateral rectus muscle, inability to elevate, depress, or adduct eye, and pupil fully dilated (the normally acting sympathetic influences are unopposed due to the absence of parasympathetic influences conveyed by the damaged parasympathetic fibers of n. III). The consensual

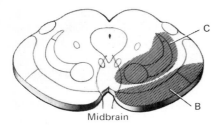

Midbrain

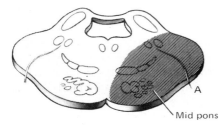

Mid pons

Figure 14.3 Sites of lesions in the pons and midbrain as described in the text. In the midpons, the lesion is located laterally (A). In the superior collicular level of the midbrain, the lesions are located in the basal region (B) and in the midbrain tegmentum (C).

light reflex to the contralateral eye is normal (Chap. 16). An *alternating hemiplegia* is a consequence of the lower motor neuron paralysis of the extraocular muscles and the upper motor neuron paralysis of the contralateral side of the body from the damage to the corticospinal tract.

The unilateral interruption of the corticobulbar and corticoreticular (indirect corticobulbar) fibers results in only minimal, if any, effects upon the muscles innervated by the cranial nerves except for the contralateral muscles of facial expression of the lower face. In general, the motor nuclei of the cranial nerves (except for the neurons of the facial nucleus innervating the lower face) receive upper motor neuron influences from both halves of the cerebrum (Chap. 9). Hence supranuclear unilateral lesions interrupting the upper motor neurons to these motor nuclei do not produce upper motor neuron paralysis of the muscles innervated by these nerves, except for the weakness of the contralateral muscles of facial expression of the lower face. In some individuals, the interruption of the upper motor neurons results in a tongue and jaw which deviate to the side contralateral to the lesion; the explanation for the observation is that these patients have few, if any, upper motor neurons originating in the ipsilateral cerebral cortex.

The bilateral, diffuse involvement of the corticobulbar and corticoreticular fibers results in a *pseudobulbar palsy*. In this syndrome there is a bilateral paralysis or weakness without atrophy of many muscles innervated by cranial nerves. The muscle groups affected control chewing, swallowing, speaking, and breathing. Unrestrained crying and laughing occur in many subjects with pseudobulbar palsy. These emotional outbursts may be related to release from influences derived from cerebral cortex and subcortical centers in the telencephalon and diencephalon.

UPPER MIDBRAIN TEGMENTUM

A unilateral lesion in the midbrain tegmentum (Fig. 14.3C) limited to the region including the fibers of the oculomotor nerve, red nucleus, superior cerebellar peduncle, medial lemniscus, and spinothalamic tract results in *Benedikt's syndrome*. The damage to the red nucleus and the fibers of the superior cerebellar peduncle (decussated dentatorubral and dentatothalamic fibers) results in such signs of cerebellar damage as coarse intention tremor, adiadochokinesis, cerebellar ataxia, and hypotonia on the contralateral side of the body (Chap. 15). Experimental evidence indicates that no signs in this syndrome are definitely attributable to a lesion of the red nucleus itself. The injury to the third cranial nerve results in a lower motor neuron paralysis of the ipsilateral extraocular muscles and in a dilated pupil (mydriasis) from absence of parasympathetic influences (see "Basal Region of the Midbrain" above). The interruption of the crossed spinothalamic tract, anterior trigeminothalamic tract, and medial lemniscus results in the loss of sense of pain, temperature, light touch, vibratory sense, pressure touch, and other discriminatory senses on the opposite side of the body and head. The retention of touch and other discriminatory senses on the contralateral side of the head may occur when the uncrossed posterior trigeminothalamic tract is intact.

Cerebellum

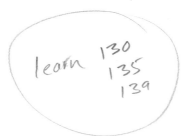

The cerebellum is located in the posterior cranial fossa inferior to the tentorium and posterior to the pons and medulla. It has essential roles in the maintenance of muscle tone and equilibrium and in phasic somatic motor activities. This suprasegmental structure functions primarily to smooth out and to synchronize the delicate and precise timing among contracting muscles of a group or groups of muscles. A patient with a cerebellar lesion is usually capable of carrying out general outlines of movements, but each movement is executed with an inadequacy of muscular coordination. The cerebellum plays no part in the perception and appreciation of conscious sensations or in intelligence.

Actually the cerebellum is a processor of sensory input of the immediate, ongoing motor activity in an organism. This sensory input, all of it on the unconscious level, is derived from the vestibular system, from the stretch receptors (neuromuscular spindles and Golgi tendon organs), and from other general sensors in the head and body. Some information is derived from the auditory and optic systems. This input is functionally integrated into the motor pathway systems and into the cerebellar feedback circuits to the cerebral cortex, vestibular system, and brainstem reticular formation.

eliminate

GROSS ANATOMY

The *cerebellum* consists of (1) an outer gray mantle, the *cortex,* (2) a *medullary core* of white matter composed of nerve fibers projecting to and from the cerebellum, and (3) *four pairs of deep cerebellar nuclei* (*nucleus fastigii, nucleus globosus, nucleus emboliformis,* and *nucleus dentatus*). The nuclei globosus and emboliformis are often called the *nucleus interpositus.* The cerebellar surface is corrugated into parallel long narrow "gyri" called *folia;* about 15 percent of the cortex is exposed to the outer surface, whereas 85 percent faces the sulcal surfaces between the folia. The cerebellum is connected to the brainstem by three cerebellar peduncles: (1) the *inferior cerebellar peduncle* is the bridge between the medulla and the cerebellum and is composed of fibers projecting both to and from the cerebellum, (2) the *middle cerebellar peduncle* is the bridge between the basilar portion of the pons and the cerebellum and is composed of fibers projecting to the cerebellum, and (3) the *superior cerebellar peduncle* is the bridge between the midbrain and the cerebellum and is composed mainly of fibers projecting from the cerebellum to the brainstem and the thalamus, and a few fibers of the anterior spinocerebellar tract projecting to the cerebellum.

The cerebellum is divided into two large bilateral hemispheres and the unpaired narrow median *vermis.* The cortex of the cerebellar hemisphere and the nucleus to which it projects (the nucleus dentatus) are grouped into the *lateral zone.* The vermal cortex and the nucleus to which it projects (the nucleus fastigii) are grouped into the *median zone.* The paravermal cortex (between vermal cortex and hemisphere cortex) and the nucleus to which it projects (the nucleus interpositus) are grouped into the *intermediate zone.*

The cerebellum may be separated into three transverse divisions (Fig. 15.1): archicerebellum (also called vestibulocerebellum or flocculonodular lobe), paleocerebellum, and neocerebellum. The phylogenetically old *archicerebellum* consists of the paired flocculi of the hemispheres and the unpaired nodulus of the vermis. This *flocculonodular lobe* is integrated with the vestibular system; it subserves a significant role in muscle tone, equilibrium, and posture through its influences on the trunk (axial) musculature. The *paleocerebellum* consists of the cerebellum rostral to the primary fissure; this *anterior lobe* is primarily associated with the proprioceptive and exteroceptive input from the head and body; it has a role in the regulation of muscle tone. The phylogenetically new *neocerebellum* consists of the cerebellum between the primary fissure and the posterolateral fissure; it includes the bulk of the hemispheres and part of the vermis. The posterolateral fissure separates the neocerebellum from the archicerebellum. The neocerebellum has a significant role in muscular coordination during phasic activities. Variations in the definition of these subdivisions are described by some authors.

e lim.

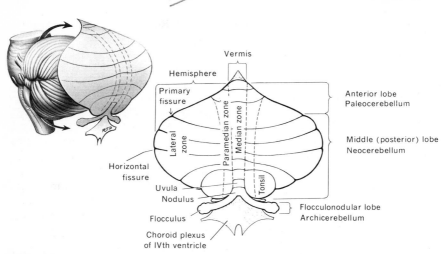

Figure 15.1 Diagram of the major subdivisions and some landmarks as viewed on the surface of the cerebellum (after surface is unfolded and laid out flat).

CEREBELLAR CORTEX (Fig. 15.2)

The *cerebellar cortex* is divided into three layers: the *molecular layer,* the middle or *Purkinje layer,* and the *granular layer.* All folia have the same neuronal organization (Fig. 15.2). The billions of cerebellar neurons are arranged and oriented as follows: (1) Each *granule cell* has a cell body and four to six short dendrites located within the granular layer; its axon projects to the molecular layer, where it bifurcates as a T into two branches which course in opposite directions parallel to the long axis of the folium (called *parallel fibers*). These axonal branches form axodendritic excitatory synapses with the dendrites of Purkinje cells, stellate cells, Golgi cells, and basket cells. (2) The *stellate cells* and *basket cells* (*inner stellate cells*) are found wholly within the molecular layer. Each of these neurons has its axon oriented at right angles to the long axis of a folium. Each stellate cell has inhibitory axodendritic synaptic connections with the dendrites of several Purkinje cells. Each basket cell has inhibitory axosomatic synaptic connections with cell bodies (basket spray endings) of several Purkinje cells. (3) Each *Golgi cell* has its dendritic tree within the molecular layer; its axon terminates as inhibitory axodendritic synapses with dendrites of granule cells within several glomeruli (see below) of the granular layer. (4) Each *Purkinje cell* has its cell body in the middle layer of the cortex; its dendritic tree arborizes into the molecular layer in a plane perpendicular to the folium, and its axon projects to form inhibitory synaptic connections with neurons in the deep cerebellar nuclei (some archicerebellar Purkinje cells have inhibitory synaptic connections

e lim

with neurons of the lateral vestibular nucleus). Recurrent axonal collaterals of each Purkinje cell have inhibitory synaptic connections with other Purkinje cells, basket cells, and Golgi cells.

INTRACEREBELLAR CIRCUITS

The *climbing fibers* (largely from inferior olivary nuclei) and *mossy fibers* (from brainstem and spinal cord nuclei) are the two types of axonal fibers conveying input directly from the spinal cord and brainstem through the cerebellar peduncles to the deep cerebellar nuclei and cerebellar cortex.

The climbing fibers form excitatory axodendritic synaptic connections with the dendritic branches of the Purkinje cells; branches from the main axon have other excitatory synaptic connections with the neurons of the deep cerebellar nuclei, basket cells, stellate cells, granule cells, and Golgi cells. The climbing fibers exert powerful excitatory influences upon the Purkinje cells,

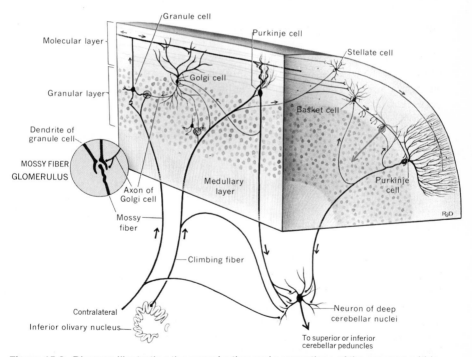

Figure 15.2 Diagram illustrating the organization and connections of the neurons within a cerebellar folium. A transverse section through a folium is represented on the right and a longitudinal section (long axis) through a folium on the left.

which, in turn, are stimulated to exert inhibitory influences upon the deep cerebellar nuclei (and the lateral vestibular nucleus).

The mossy fibers pass through the cerebellar peduncles, branch profusely, and terminate in mosslike excrescences in the cerebellar glomeruli of the granular layer. A *glomerulus* (Fig. 15.2) is a synaptic complex formed by (1) the excitatory synapse between a mossy fiber (or climbing fiber) excrescence and a dendrite of a granule cell and (2) several inhibitory axodendritic synapses between Golgi cells and a granule cell. In turn, the granule cell conveys excitatory influences via parallel fibers to the dendrites of Purkinje cells (called "crossing-over synapses"), stellate cells, basket cells, and Golgi cells. In turn, the stellate cells and basket cells exert inhibitory influences upon Purkinje cells and Golgi cells; the latter convey inhibitory influences to the glomeruli.

The output of the cerebellar cortex (Purkinje cells) is inhibitory to the neurons of the deep cerebellar nuclei (and lateral vestibular nucleus), whereas the output of the deep cerebellar nuclei is known to be of an excitatory nature. The precise mechanisms for regulating the cerebellar output are not known in detail. Collaterals from the mossy fibers and climbing fibers are presumed to convey facilitatory influences to the deep cerebellar nuclei. The degree of inhibition exerted via the stellate cells and basket cells on the Purkinje cells determines the responsiveness of the Purkinje cells when they are stimulated by the excitatory influences from the climbing fibers. With the deep cerebellar nuclei receiving both excitatory and inhibitory influences, current thought indicates that facilitatory influences usually predominate over the inhibitory influences and thereby maintain tonic discharges of excitatory impulses to the nuclei of the brainstem and thalamus involved with influencing motor activity.

GENERAL CEREBELLAR CIRCUITRY

Input to the Cerebellum

There are approximately three times as many cerebellar afferent fibers as cerebellar efferent fibers.

The *inferior cerebellar peduncle* (*restiform body*) is composed of fibers of the posterior spinocerebellar tract, cuneocerebellar tract, rostral spinocerebellar tract, reticulocerebellar fibers, olivocerebellar fibers, and trigeminocerebellar fibers. The *juxtarestiform body* (bundle of fibers on medial aspect of the inferior cerebellar peduncle) has vestibulocerebellar fibers (Chap. 13). The posterior spinocerebellar, cuneocerebellar, and rostral cerebellar tracts convey influences from the stretch and exteroceptive receptors of the body via the spinal cord to the anterior lobe of the cerebellum (Chap. 8). The reticulocerebellar fibers project from the lateral reticular nucleus of the medulla (input to this nucleus is from spinal cord, red nucleus, and cerebellar

learn

fastigial nucleus) and paramedian nuclei of medulla largely as uncrossed components to the anterior lobe and vermis. The olivocerebellar fibers originate in the contralateral inferior olivary nucleus of the medulla and terminate in all cortical areas of the cerebellum. The accessory olivary nuclei project to the vermis, and the principal olivary nucleus projects to a cerebellar hemisphere. Input to the inferior olivary nuclei is derived from the cerebral cortex, brainstem reticular nuclei, and red nucleus. The *inferior olivary nucleus* is presumed to be the major source of climbing fibers of the cerebellum. The trigeminocerebellar fibers convey influences from stretch and exteroceptive receptors of the head. Primary fibers from the vestibular nerve and secondary fibers from vestibular nuclei pass, as vestibulocerebellar fibers, through the juxtarestiform body before terminating in the cortex of the flocculonodular lobe and adjacent cortex (referred to as *vestibulocerebellum*) and the fastigial nuclei (Chap. 13).

The *middle cerebellar peduncle (brachium pontis)* is composed of crossed pontocerebellar fibers projecting from the pontine nuclei to the neocerebellum and paleocerebellum. This tract is involved with conveying influences from the cerebral cortex via the corticopontine tract (see below under "Feedback Loops").

The *superior cerebellar peduncle (brachium conjunctivum)* contains fibers of the anterior spinocerebellar tract, which terminate in the anterior lobe. (See "NA Pathways from the Locus Ceruleus," p. 99, and Fig. 11.6.)

Output from the Cerebellum

The influences from the cerebellum on motor coordination are mediated through indirect pathways; no direct cerebellospinal pathways are present.

The outflow through the juxtarestiform body includes (1) crossed and uncrossed fastigiobulbar fibers from the fastigial nuclei to the vestibular nuclei and reticular nuclei of the pons and medulla, and (2) some direct fibers from the vestibulocerebellum (flocculonodular lobe) to the vestibular nuclei. Some fibers from the fastigial nuclei hook around the rostral aspect of the superior cerebellar peduncle as the *uncinate* (hooked) fasciculus before passing through the juxtarestiform body. Each fastigial nucleus receives input from the vestibular nuclei and archicerebellum.

The *superior cerebellar peduncle* consists primarily of efferent fibers from the dentate, emboliform, and globose nuclei (designated collectively as *dentato-*) as the dentatorubral, dentatothalamic, and dentatoreticular fibers. The entire outflow crosses over in the lower midbrain as the decussation of the superior cerebellar peduncle. Most fibers from the dentate nucleus project rostrally to the ventral lateral thalamic nucleus and intralaminar thalamic nuclei, with some fibers terminating in the rostral third of the nucleus ruber; other fibers project caudally as the *descendens of the superior cerebellar peduncle* to the brainstem reticular nuclei (reticulotegmental nucleus). The globose and emboliform nuclei project mainly to the caudal two-thirds of the nucleus ruber and to brainstem reticular nuclei.

Feedback Loops

The cerebellum is integrated into a number of circuits and feedback loops.

The *cerebrocerebellar loop* (Fig. 15.3) interconnects the cerebrum with the cerebellum. Volitional movements initiated in the cerebral cortex probably utilize this feedback loop to modulate coordinated movements. The core of this circuit includes, in order, (1) the corticopontine tracts (from widespread areas of the cerebral cortex to the ipsilateral pontine nuclei), (2) the crossed

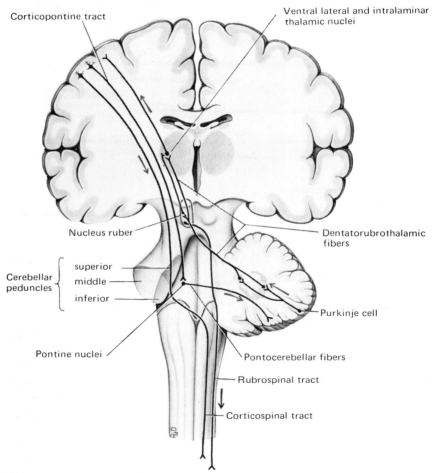

Figure 15.3 Cerebellar (neocerebellar) connections with the cerebral cortex, thalamus, and some brainstem nuclei.

elim.

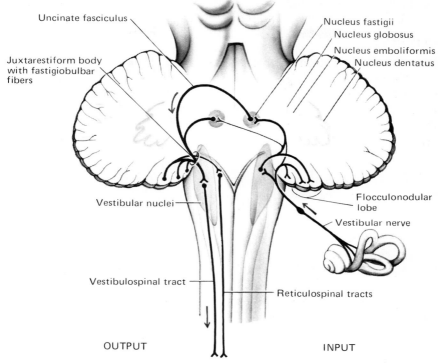

Uncinate fasciculus

Juxtarestiform body
with fastigiobulbar
fibers

Nucleus fastigii
Nucleus globosus
Nucleus emboliformis
Nucleus dentatus

Vestibular nuclei

Flocculonodular
lobe

Vestibular nerve

Vestibulospinal tract

Reticulospinal tracts

OUTPUT   INPUT

Figure 15.4 Cerebellar connections of the vestibulocerebellum (archicerebellum and fastigial nucleus) with the vestibular nerve and vestibular nuclei.

pontocerebellar fibers to the contralateral neocerebellar cortex and deep cerebellar nuclei, (3) the Purkinje cell routes to the deep cerebellar nuclei, and (4) the decussating dentatorubrothalamic cortical pathway terminating in the motor cerebral cortex (area 4). This loop exerts influences upon descending motor pathways from the cerebral cortex.

The *vestibular archicerebellar loop* (Fig. 15.4) includes (1) the input limb from the vestibular nerve and vestibular nuclei to the archicerebellar cortex and fastigial nuclei, and (2) the output limb from the vestibulocerebellum including nucleus fastigii, through the juxtarestiform body to the vestibular nuclei and reticular nuclei of the brainstem. This loop exerts influences through the vestibulospinal and reticulospinal tracts upon spinal motor activity (Chap. 9).

The *brainstem nuclei cerebellar loop* is the sequence (1) from lower brainstem reticular nuclei and inferior olivary nucleus via the reticulocerebellar and olivocerebellar fibers to the cerebellar cortex and deep cerebellar nuclei and, to complete the loop, (2) via the dentatorubroreticular fibers and _elim_

descendens of the superior cerebellar peduncle to brainstem reticular nuclei. This loop exerts influences through the rubrospinal and reticulospinal pathways upon spinal motor activity (Chap. 9).

FUNCTIONAL ROLE OF THE CEREBELLUM

The cerebellum is the great modulator subserving the coordination of groups of muscles, especially the agonist and the antagonist muscles (*synergy*). It smooths the ongoing actions of muscle groups by delicately regulating and grading muscle tensions. Acting as a servomechanism in a negative-feedback system, the cerebellum functions to prevent oscillations (*tremor*) during motion and thereby maintains stability in movements. A large lesion of the cerebellum releases other processing centers of the nervous system from cerebellar influences. The release phenomena which result illustrate the loss of the effects of the negative-feedback system. In moving the upper extremity to touch an object with the tip of a finger there is an intention tremor—the extremity oscillates in a series of rhythmic movements as it approaches the object. This resembles the automatic-pilot control system, in which each correction is followed by a small overshoot. In normal cerebellar activity the negative-feedback activity reduces the overshoot to insignificance.

CEREBELLAR DYSFUNCTION

Lesions of the cerebellum, its input fibers, or its output fibers result in symptoms which are actually the result of the activity of noncerebellar centers (e.g., ventral lateral nucleus of thalamus). These centers are released from cerebellar influences; the resulting symptoms are expressions of release phenomena.

Unilateral cerebellar lesions have *homolateral* effects. The symptoms are expressed on the same side of the body because the pathways from the cerebellum decussate and integrate with pathway systems that, in turn, cross over to the side of the original cerebellar output to exert their effects. For example, one side of the cerebellum projects via the crossed dentatorubrothalamocortical pathway to the contralateral nucleus ruber and cerebral cortex. In turn, the rubrospinal and corticospinal tracts are crossed, descending pathways. In effect, the cerebellum exerts its influences through a double crossing of (1) the ascending fibers of the decussating superior cerebellar peduncle and (2) the decussating descending rubrospinal and corticospinal tracts.

Lesions of the cerebellum result in disturbances expressed as a *constellation* of symptoms and neurologic signs (noted below). Small lesions may produce no symptoms or only transient symptoms, whereas large lesions produce severe symptoms. The cerebellar cortex possesses a good margin of physiologic safety; with time the neurologic symptoms attenuate, and the resulting compensation markedly reduces the severity of the deficits. Atten-

learn

uation of symptoms is not likely to occur following lesions of the deep cerebellar nuclei or their axons.

Neocerebellar Lesions

With neocerebellar lesions, the tendon reflexes are diminished (*hypotonia*); this effect is expressed as a pendular knee jerk that swings freely back and forth. Muscles tire easily (*asthenia*). The horizontally extended upper extremity gradually drifts downward when the eyes are closed because the proprioceptive sense is not being properly used. *Asynergia,* or loss of muscular coordination, is expressed by jerky, puppetlike movements including the decomposition of movement, dysmetria, past pointing, and adiadochokinesis. The *decomposition of movement* is the breaking up of a movement into its component parts; instead of a smooth, coordinated flow of movement in bringing the tip of the finger of the extended upper extremity to the nose, each joint of the shoulder, elbow, wrist, and finger may flex independently (puppetlike) in an almost mechanical fashion. *Dysmetria,* or the inability to gauge or measure distances accurately, results in the overshooting of an intended goal by consistent pointing toward the lesion side of the object (*past pointing*). *Adiadochokinesis* is the impairment of the ability to execute alternating and repetitive movements such as supination and pronation of the forearm in rapid succession with equal excursions. The *intention* or *action tremor* is expressed during the execution of a voluntary movement. It is absent or diminished during rest. These tremors are particularly noted at the end of the movement (*terminal tremor*). The ataxic gait, or the asynergic activity elicited during walking, is a staggering movement resembling that of drunkenness. The ataxia is due to incoordination of the trunk and proximal girdle muscles. A tendency to veer or to fall to the side of the lesion is apparent. To counteract the unsteadiness, the patient will stand or walk with legs far apart (broad-base stance).

A *scanning speech,* or *dysarthria,* is the result of the incoordination of the muscles used in speaking. The speech is hesitating, slurred, and explosive in quality, with a telegram-staccato pace (pauses in the wrong places).

Archicerebellar Lesions

Lesions of the flocculonodular lobe may result in ataxia of the trunk muscles without any signs of tremor or hypotonia. Children with nodular lobe tumors have a tendency to fall backward, sway from side to side, and walk with a wide base and an ataxic gait. They may be unable to maintain an upright balance.

Paleocerebellar Lesions

No definite data are available to define the symptoms of a paleocerebellar lesion in man. An effect on muscle tone accompanied by an ataxic gait is probable.

Chapter 16

Visual System

Learn whole chapter

Man lives primarily in a visual world. Light waves from objects in the environment are refracted by the nonadjustable transparent cornea of the eye and are further refracted and inverted by the adjustable lens before passing through the retina where the transduction takes place in the rod cells (rods) and cone cells (cones). The amount of light entering the eye is regulated by the smooth muscles in the iris diaphragm, which controls the size of the pupil (see "Light Reflexes" below). The thickness of the lens is adjusted by the smooth muscles in the ciliary body (see "Accommodation Reflex" below).

The retinofugal projections from the eye include (1) the visual pathway to the visual cortex, (2) the pathway to the superior colliculus with relays to the visual cortex, pulvinar, and posterior thalamus, and (3) the circuits involved with several reflexes including the light and the accommodation reflexes.

VISUAL PATHWAY

The environment viewed by the eyes is called the *visual field*. The light waves in the visual field stimulate the retinal receptors, which initiate the neural activities relayed by the visual pathway to the cerebral cortex. This visual pathway comprises (1) neurons of the retina, (2) retinogeniculate projections via fibers in the optic nerve, chiasma, and tract terminating in the lateral geniculate body of the thalamus, (3) geniculostriate tract (geniculocalcarine tract, optic radiation) to the primary visual cortex (striate cortex, area 17) on the upper and lower banks of the calcarine sulcus, and (4) visual cortical association areas (areas 18 and 19). The processing sites in this pathway are the *retina, lateral geniculate body*, and *visual cortical areas* (Fig. 16.1).

Retina

The retina of each eye is conventionally divided into a temporal (lateral) hemiretina and a nasal (medial) hemiretina by a vertical line passing through the center of the *macula lutea*, a 3-mm circular area of the retina located near the posterior pole of the eye. These *hemiretinas* may be subdivided, in turn, into upper and lower quadrants by a horizontal line passing through the macula lutea. The retina is further subdivided by three concentric circles (with macula as the center) into a small macular area, a pericentral (paramacular) area, and a peripheral (monocular) area. The projections from the "spots" of the retina through the visual pathways are retinotopically organized.

The action of the lens on the projections from the visual fields (environment projected upon retina) produces an inverted (upside down) and a reversed (left for right) image on the retina. Hence the temporal visual field is projected to the nasal hemiretina, the nasal visual field to the temporal hemiretina, the upper visual field to the lower hemiretina, and so on. Without changing the fixation of an eye, the lateral peripheral area of its visual field—called a *monocular crescent*—is seen by only one eye. The rest of the visual field is seen by both eyes.

The light receptors in each eye include more than 100 million rods and 7 million cones. The transduction of light as a photochemical reaction with the photopigments and the initiation of the receptor potential takes place in the outer segment of each rod (or cone); here the role of light is completed. The retina—actually a mobile portion of the brain—is composed of rods and cones, bipolar cells, horizontal cells, amacrine cells, and ganglion cells, where the complex transformations take place. The macula lutea of the retina is in direct line with the visual axis; the *fovea centralis* is a depression in the macula where vision is sharpest and color vision is optimal.

Each of the 1 million ganglion cells in each retina receives its stimulation

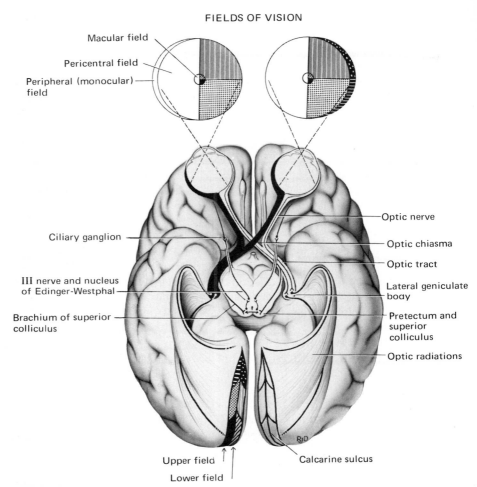

FIELDS OF VISION

Macular field

Pericentral field

Peripheral (monocular) field

Optic nerve

Ciliary ganglion

Optic chiasma

Optic tract

III nerve and nucleus of Edinger-Westphal

Lateral geniculate body

Brachium of superior colliculus

Pretectum and superior colliculus

Optic radiations

Upper field

Lower field

Calcarine sulcus

Figure 16.1 Diagram illustrating the visual pathways from the retina to the lateral geniculate bodies and to the primary visual cortex. The projection to the tectum in the midbrain is indicated.

from a spot in the environment. This cell's eye view of the environment is called the *receptor field* (*center-surround*) for that cell. It is a small circle composed of either an *on* excitatory center (hole in doughnut) and an annular *off* inhibitory surround (doughnut) or an *off* center and an *on* surround. As a result of the interactions between centers and their surrounds, the retinal ganglion cells relay signals concerning the contrast between the intensity of the illumination in the center as compared with that in the surround. In a sense each retina is a mosaic of 1 million ganglion cells which relays 1 million center-surround receptor field transformations via its axons to the lateral geniculate body of the thalamus.

Optic Nerve, Chiasma, and Tract

The optic nerve emerges from the eye at the cribriform plate (*optic disk, blind spot*). The *axons of the ganglion cells* of the retinas pass in a retinotopic order through the optic nerves, chiasma, and tracts before terminating in the lateral geniculate bodies (and in the midbrain tectum and pretectum). The fibers from the *temporal hemiretinas* project to the ipsilateral lateral geniculate bodies (they do not decussate in the optic chiasm). The fibers from the *nasal hemiretinas* project to the contralateral lateral geniculate bodies (fibers decussate in the optic chiasm). In effect, the temporal hemiretina of one eye and the nasal hemiretina of the other eye (hemiretinas which view the same visual fields) project to the same lateral geniculate body. However, the projections from the hemiretinas are separate (no overlap), with the fibers from each temporal hemiretina terminating on neurons in laminae II, III, and V and from each nasal hemiretina on neurons in laminae I, IV, and VI of the lateral geniculate body. The influences from the right visual fields to each eye are projected to the left geniculate body and those from the left visual fields to each eye to the right geniculate body. Each geniculate neuron responds to stimulation from one eye only. The receptive fields of the neurons in the lateral geniculate body elicit similar responses as those of the retinal ganglion cells—the doughnut effect of a center with an annular surround.

Optic Radiation and the Visual Cortex

The fibers from the lateral geniculate body pass in a retinotopic organization through the retrolenticular portion of the internal capsule and continue posteriorly as the *optic radiation* along the lateral aspect of the lateral ventricle before terminating in laminae III and IV of the primary visual cortex (Chap. 22). Fibers in the upper half of the optic radiation convey influences from the upper hemiretinas and those in the lower half of the optic radiation from the lower hemiretinas. Fibers from the lower peripheral retinas arch through the temporal lobe, as the temporal *Meyer's loop*, before coursing posteriorly.

The *primary visual cortex* (area 17) is organized into "physiologically" defined columns extending from the pial surface to the white matter. The act of binocular fusion of the receptor fields from the two hemiretinas occurs within laminae of these columns other than lamina IV. The primary visual cortex is organized such that the projections from each upper hemiretina terminate within area 17 of the cuneus and those from each lower hemiretina terminate within area 17 of the lingual gyrus. The macular, pericentral, and monocular peripheral retinal areas are represented in the posterior, intermediate, and anterior portions of area 17, respectively. The large caudal cortical representation of macular vision is associated with the sharp visual acuity monitored by the macula. The pericentral retinal area, an area registering minimal visual acuity, is represented by a small cortical area.

Influences from area 17 (visual area I) are relayed to area 18 (visual area II) and area 19 (visual area III); these areas are small, mirror-image representations of area 17. Areas 18 and 19 (but not area 17) are reciprocally connected (1) with their counterparts on the contralateral hemisphere via fibers passing through the corpus callosum and (2) with the pulvinar of the thalamus.

The input to the cortex from the circular geniculate fields is transformed into linear and rectangular fields. On the basis of their receptive fields, the cortical neurons have been classified as simple, complex, and hypercomplex cells. The *simple cells* are detectors of straight lines, each having a correct orientation and position in the retina. The *complex cells* are detectors of straight lines, each having a correct orientation but a variable position in the retina, while the *hypercomplex cells* are detectors of angled and curved lines. Area 17 has simple and complex neurons, and areas 18 and 19 contain complex and hypercomplex neurons.

The superior colliculus (actually a laminated cortical structure), the pulvinar, and the posterior thalamus are in an as yet unknown way integrated into the process of visual perception. The colliculus has been implicated in the detection of movement.

REFLEX PATHWAYS

Light Reflexes (Fig. 16.2)

When a bright light is directed into an unfixed eye, the pupils of both eyes constrict following the contraction of the constrictor muscles of the iris. The response in the stimulated eye is called the *direct light response,* and that in the unstimulated eye is called the *consensual light response.* The sequence and course of neurons in this arc are as follows: (1) Retinofugal fibers of the ganglion cells of each eye pass through the optic nerve, chiasma, tract, and brachium of the superior colliculus before terminating in both sides of the pretectum of the midbrain (some fibers cross and some do not cross as they pass through the optic chiasma). (2) The two halves of the pretectum are interconnected by fibers passing through the posterior commissure. (3) Axons of pretectal neurons project to the accessory oculomotor nuclei of Edinger-Westphal of the same and opposite sides. (4) The preganglionic parasympathetic neurons have fibers which pass through the IIIrd nerve and terminate by synapsing in the ciliary ganglion with postganglionic neurons. (5) The latter innervate the constrictor smooth muscle of the iris. The consensual

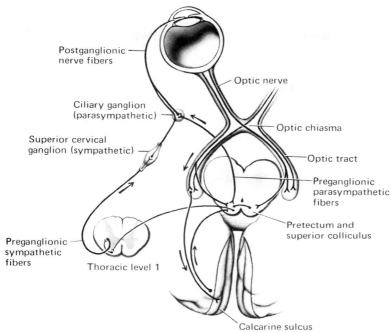

Postganglionic nerve fibers

Optic nerve

Ciliary ganglion (parasympathetic)

Optic chiasma

Superior cervical ganglion (sympathetic)

Optic tract

Preganglionic parasympathetic fibers

Pretectum and superior colliculus

Preganglionic sympathetic fibers

Thoracic level 1

Calcarine sulcus

Figure 16.2 Diagram illustrating the light reflex pathways (pupillary reflex) and the pathway associated with accommodation.

light reflex influences the unstimulated eye by fibers that cross in the optic chiasma and the posterior commissure of the midbrain. These reflexes are carried out unconsciously, without any cortical involvement.

Accommodation Reflex (Fig. 16.2)

The adjustments of the lens by the action of the ciliary body to bring an object into focus are known as accommodation. Unlike the light reflexes, the accommodation reflex includes the visual cortex; an individual does exert some control in selecting the object brought into focus. Visual influences from the eye are relayed via the visual pathways to the visual cortex. Neurons in the visual areas have axons which descend through the optic radiation to the superior colliculus of the midbrain. In turn, collicular interneurons stimulate the preganglionic parasympathetic neurons of the accessory oculomotor nucleus of Edinger-Westphal which, after passing through the IIIrd nerve, synapse with postganglionic parasympathetic neurons in the ciliary ganglion. These neurons innervate the smooth muscles in the ciliary body, which regulates the tension on the lens.

Accommodation-Convergence Reaction

Immediately after the eyes are shifted from a distant object to a near one (near-sight vision), several activities occur. The lens thickens in order to bring the object into focus by accommodation. The eyes converge as the medial recti muscles contract. The pupils constrict to increase the definition of the image.

Pupillary Dilatation

Descending sympathetic pathways pass through the brainstem and anterior half of the spinal cord before terminating with preganglionic neurons of the intermediolateral cell column in C8 and T1 spinal levels. The preganglionic fibers ascend through the sympathetic chain and synapse with postganglionic

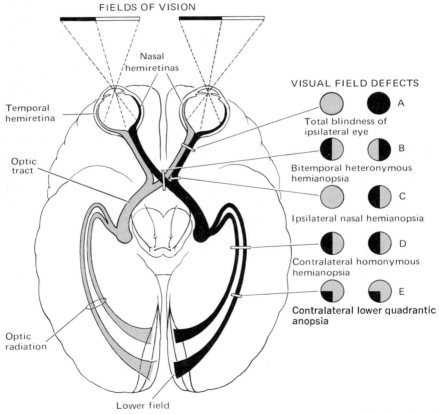

Figure 16.3 Diagram of some common lesions at various levels within the visual pathways. The corresponding *visual field defects* are represented on the right side.

sympathetic neurons, which course along branches of the internal carotid artery before they innervate the pupillary dilator fibers in the iris.

LESIONS WITHIN VISUAL PATHWAYS (Fig. 16.3)

Impairment of a small area of the retina results in a blind spot (*scotoma*) in that eye. The *optic disk* is a natural blind spot; it contains no rods and cones. The complete interruption of the optic nerve results in permanent blindness in one eye (Fig. 16.3A). However, this blind eye can still accommodate and exhibit the consensual light reflex because the normal eye activates the reflex arcs to the blind eye.

A *midline lesion of the optic chiasma* (pressure from a tumor of the pituitary gland) may interrupt the decussating fibers from both eyes (Fig. 16.3B). This results in blindness in the nasal half of the retina (the temporal half of the visual field of each eye); it is called *bitemporal heteronymous hemianopsia (hemianopia)*. Damage to the nondecussating fibers on one (right) side of the optic chiasma results in a *right nasal hemianopsia* (Fig. 16.3C), i.e., blindness in the temporal half of the retina (nasal half of the visual field of one eye). The complete interruption of the optic tract, lateral geniculate body, optic radiations, or entire primary visual cortex on one (right) side results in a *contralateral homonymous hemianopsia,* or blindness in the field of vision on the opposite (left) side of the lesion (Fig. 16.3D). Visual defects limited to a single visual field are *homonymous*, whereas those located in both fields are *heteronymous.* Partial lesions produce partial defects in the fields of vision. A lesion of the entire cuneus (includes entire primary visual cortex above the calcarine sulcus) on one side results in *contralateral lower quadrantic anopsia* (Fig. 16.3E), because pathways from the upper temporal quadrant of the ipsilateral retina and upper nasal quadrant of the contralateral retina are interrupted.

Autonomic Nervous System

The functional activity of the nervous system is usually expressed by the contraction (or relaxation) of muscles and the secretion of glands. These actions are mediated through the somatic motor system and the visceral motor system (autonomic nervous system). The *somatic motor system* innervates the voluntary (skeletal, striated) muscles, whereas the *autonomic nervous system* influences the activities of involuntary (smooth) muscles, cardiac (heart) muscle, and glands. The autonomic nervous system is often called the *general visceral efferent system* or *vegetative motor system* because the effectors are associated with the visceral systems (e.g., cardiovascular, digestive, and respiratory systems) over which only a minimal, if any, direct conscious control can be exerted.

THE SOMATIC AND AUTONOMIC NERVOUS SYSTEMS

The basic role of the somatic motor system is to regulate the coordinated muscular activities associated with the maintenance of posture and with phasic locomotor movements; these expressions are related to adjustments to the external environment. The general role of the autonomic nervous system is to influence those visceral activities which are directed toward maintaining a relatively stable internal environment within the body. For example, the maintenance of (1) the blood pressure commensurate with the demands of the organism and (2) a constant body temperature are functional expressions of the activity of the autonomic nervous system. These two systems are not independent; they do interact. For example, with a drop in body temperature, the somatic nervous system responds by generating heat through contraction of voluntary muscles, and the autonomic nervous system stimulates the constriction of cutaneous blood vessels to reduce the heat loss by radiation. In general the somatic nervous system reacts rapidly to stimulation, whereas the autonomic nervous system responds with a greater time lag.

The two systems differ significantly with reference to the anatomic organization of the final neuronal linkage between the central nervous system and the peripherally located effectors. The somatic motor system has a *one-neuron linkage* (alpha and gamma motor neurons) and the autonomic nervous system has a *two-neuron linkage* (Fig. 17.1). From its cell body in the

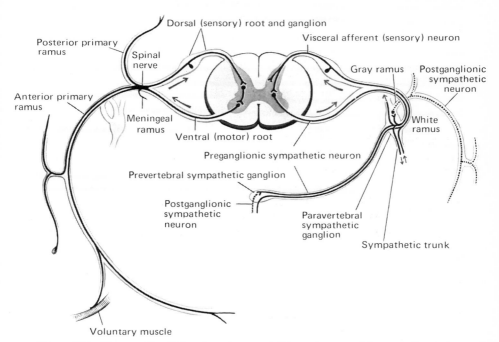

Figure 17.1 Diagram illustrating the neurons of (A) a reflex arc of the somatic nervous system on the left, and (B) a visceral reflex arc of the sympathetic nervous system on the right. The spinal somatic reflex arc is described in Chap. 5.

brainstem or spinal cord, each somatic lower motor neuron has an axon which courses through a cranial or spinal nerve to make synaptic connections (at motor end-plates) with voluntary muscle fibers (Chap. 9). In contrast, the first neuron of the autonomic nervous system, called a *preganglionic neuron*, originates in the brainstem or spinal cord and has an axon which courses through a cranial or peripheral nerve and terminates by synapsing with a second neuron (or neurons) located in an autonomic ganglion outside the central nervous system. This second neuron, called a *postganglionic neuron*, has an axon which extends peripherally to terminate in endings associated with smooth muscles, cardiac muscle, or glands.

The autonomic nervous system is conventionally considered to be a motor system—the general visceral efferent motor system.

SUBDIVISIONS OF THE AUTONOMIC NERVOUS SYSTEM

The autonomic nervous system is divided into two systems, the sympathetic system and the parasympathetic system. The *sympathetic system* stimulates those activities which are mobilized by the organism during emergency and stress situations—the so-called "fight, fright, and flight" responses. These include the acceleration of the rate and force of the heartbeat, increase in the concentration of blood sugar, and increase in blood pressure. In contrast, the *parasympathetic system* stimulates those activities associated with conservation and restoration of body resources of the organism. These include decrease in the rate of the heartbeat and the rise in gastrointestinal activities associated with increased digestion and absorption of food.

The sympathetic system is also called the *thoracolumbar* or *adrenergic system* because (1) its preganglionic fibers emerge from all thoracic and upper two lumbar levels (T1 through L2) and (2) the neurosecretory transmitter released by the postganglionic fibers is norepinephrine (noradrenalin). The parasympathetic system is also called the *craniosacral* or *cholinergic system* because (1) its preganglionic fibers emerge with cranial nerves III, VII, IX, X, the cranial root of XI, and at sacral spinal levels S3 through S4, and (2) the neurosecretory transmitter released by the postganglionic fibers is acetylcholine.

SYMPATHETIC (THORACOLUMBAR) SYSTEM (Fig. 17.2)

Preganglionic fibers of the sympathetic system originate from cell bodies located in the intermediolateral nucleus of lamina VII which extends from spinal levels T1 through L2. These fibers pass successively through the ventral roots—where they are referred to as the *thoracolumbar outflow*—of the spinal nerves, the white rami communicantes (branches of the spinal nerves), and the sympathetic trunk; after branching, they terminate by

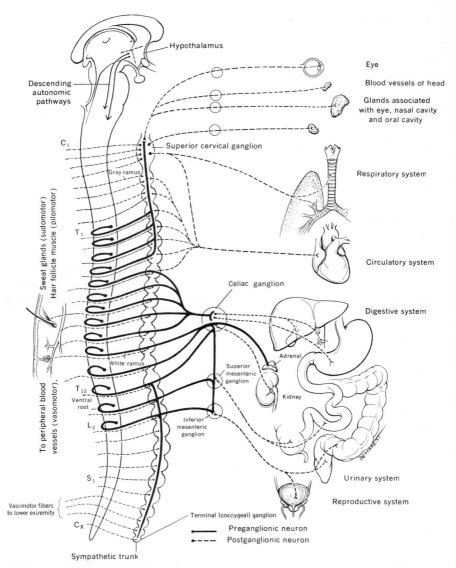

Hypothalamus

Eye

Blood vessels of head

Glands associated
with eye, nasal cavity
and oral cavity

Descending
autonomic
pathways

C_1

Superior cervical ganglion

Gray ramus

Respiratory system

T_1

Circulatory system

Celiac ganglion

Digestive system

Adrenal

White ramus

Superior
mesenteric
ganglion

T_{12}
Ventral
root

Kidney

L_2

Inferior
mesenteric
ganglion

S_1

Urinary system

Reproductive system

Vasomotor fibers
to lower extremity

C_x

Terminal (coccygeal) ganglion

Sweat glands (sudomotor)
Hair follicle muscle (pilomotor)

To peripheral blood
vessels (vasomotor)

Preganglionic neuron
Postganglionic neuron

Sympathetic trunk

Figure 17.2 Diagram of the sympathetic (thoracolumbar) division of the autonomic nervous system.

synapsing within either (1) the ganglia of the paravertebral ganglia of the sympathetic chain or (2) the prevertebral (collateral) ganglia. The paravertebral ganglia of the *sympathetic chain* (trunk), which are located along the centra of the vertebral column from the upper cervical through coccygeal levels, receive their input exclusively from the thoracolumbar sympathetic outflow. The paired sympathetic chains meet in the midline in a terminal ganglion on the coccyx, called the *ganglion impar* or coccygeal ganglion. The prevertebral ganglia are located in the abdomen adjacent to the abdominal aorta and its main branches—the celiac, aorticorenal, superior mesenteric, and inferior mesenteric ganglia (derived from T6 through L2 spinal levels).

The postganglionic fibers from cells in the paravertebral ganglia pass via (1) the gray rami communicantes and the spinal nerves before terminating in association with the sweat glands and the smooth muscles of blood vessels and hair (erector pili muscles) of the body wall and extremities and (2) small nerves and perivascular plexuses to the visceral structures of the head, neck, and thorax (e.g., pupillary dilator muscle, heart, bronchioles). The postganglionic fibers from cells in the prevertebral ganglia form the perivascular plexuses innervating the abdominal and pelvic viscera. In general, the sympathetic outflow is distributed as follows: T1 to T5 to the head and neck, T1 and T2 to the eye, T2 to T6 to the heart and lungs, T6 and L2 to the abdominal viscera, and L1 to L2 to the urinary, genital, and lower digestive systems. The *neurotransmitter* released by the preganglionic nerve terminals is *acetylcholine*, which is deactivated rapidly by *cholinesterase;* that released by the postganglionic nerve terminals is *norepinephrine* (*noradrenalin, levarterenol*), which is deactivated slowly by *monoamine oxidase* (*MAO*) and *catechol-o-methyl transferase* (*COMT*) or taken up again by the nerve terminals. The MAO is located intracellularly, while the COMT is found extracellularly.

Adrenal Gland

The cells of the medulla of the adrenal gland are actually specialized postganglionic neurons. Preganglionic cholinergic fibers from T6 to T9 stimulate the adrenal chromaffin cells to release both norepinephrine and epinephrine into the circulatory system, which distributes these neurosecretions throughout the body. The adrenal medulla–released transmitters act in conjunction with norepinephrine released by the sympathetic postganglionic fibers.

Systemic Effects of Sympathetic Innervation

The sympathetic system is structurally and functionally organized to exert its influences over widespread body regions or even the entire body for sustained periods of time. Each preganglionic neuron has a relatively short axon which synapses with many postganglionic neurons, each of which has a long branching axon forming numerous neuroeffector junctions over a wide area. The widespread and sustained sympathetic effects are due to the slow deactivation of norepinephrine and to the systemic distribution of norepinephrine and epinephrine released by the adrenal medulla.

PARASYMPATHETIC (CRANIOSACRAL) SYSTEM
(Fig. 17.3)

The cranial portion of the parasympathetic system is associated with (1) four cranial nerves (ns. III, VII, IX, and X) that supply the parasympathetic innervation to the head and thoracic and most of the abdominal viscera, and (2) the sacral spinal cord that supplies the innervation to the lower abdominal and pelvic viscera. The body wall and the extremities do not have a para- sympathetic innervation. From cell bodies in the accessory oculomotor nucleus of Edinger-Westphal (midbrain), preganglionic fibers pass via the IIIrd cranial nerve and terminate in the ciliary ganglion with postganglionic neurons which innervate the sphincter (constrictor) muscles of the pupil and ciliary muscles involved with accommodation (focusing of lens of eye). From cell bodies in the superior salivatory nucleus, preganglionic fibers pass via the VIIth cranial nerve and terminate in the pterygopalatine and submandibular ganglia with postganglionic neurons which innervate numerous glands in the head including lacrimal, submandibular, and sublingual glands and glands of the nasal, oral, and pharyngeal cavities. From cell bodies in the inferior salivatory nucleus, preganglionic fibers pass via the IXth cranial nerve and terminate in the otic ganglion with postganglionic neurons which innervate the parotid gland. From preganglionic cells in the dorsal vagal nucleus, preganglionic fibers pass via the Xth cranial nerve and synapse within terminal ganglia (located adjacent to or within visceral organs) with post- ganglionic neurons which innervate the viscera of the thorax and abdomen (e.g., heart, lungs, and gastrointestinal tract). The sacral portion of the parasympathetic system originates from cell bodies in the gray matter of sacral levels 2 to 4; these preganglionic neurons pass via the pelvic splanchnic nerves to synapse in terminal ganglia with postganglionic neurons which innervate the lower abdominal and pelvic viscera (colon distal to left colic flexure, urinary, and genital viscera). The sacral parasympathetic outflow is involved with the "mechanisms of emptying"—urination and defecation.

In general, the parasympathetic system has preganglionic fibers with long axons which synapse with a few postganglionic fibers with short axons. The neurotransmitter secretion at the terminals of both the preganglionic and postganglionic neurons is *acetylcholine*.

Systemic Effects of Parasympathetic Innervation

The parasympathetic system is primarily organized to respond to a specific stimulus in localized and discrete regions transiently for short durations. Each preganglionic neuron, a long axon synapsing with a few postganglionic neurons with short axons, exerts influences over a small area. The rapid deactivation of acetylcholine by cholinesterase restricts the time course over which a specific quantity of acetylcholine is effective.

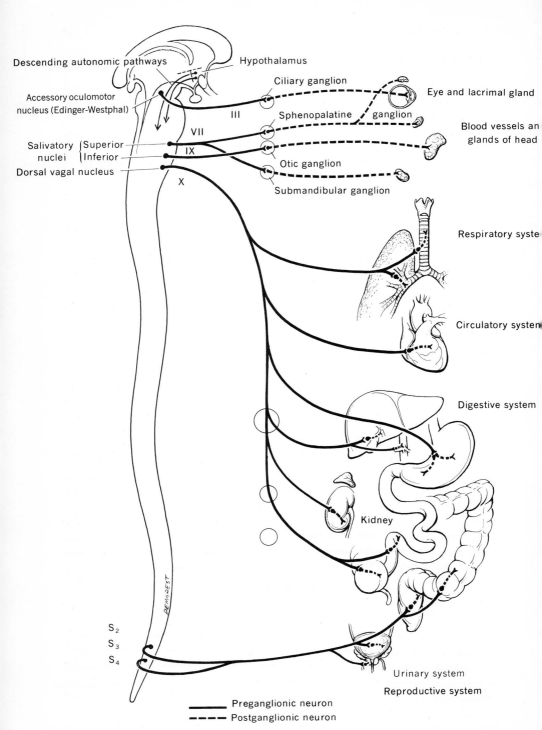

Descending autonomic pathways

Hypothalamus

Accessory oculomotor
nucleus (Edinger-Westphal)

Ciliary ganglion

Eye and lacrimal gland

III

Sphenopalatine   ganglion

Salivatory ⎰Superior
nuclei   ⎱Inferior

VII

Blood vessels an
glands of head

IX

Dorsal vagal nucleus

Otic ganglion

X

Submandibular ganglion

Respiratory syste

Circulatory system

Digestive system

Kidney

S_2
S_3
S_4

Urinary system

Reproductive system

——— Preganglionic neuron
- - - - Postganglionic neuron

Figure 17.3 Diagram of the parasympathetic (craniosacral) division of the autonomic nervous system.

DESCENDING PATHWAYS

The stimuli influencing the activity of the preganglionic neurons of the autonomic nervous system are derived from a variety of sources. Much input is conveyed from somatic and visceral sensory receptors via afferent fibers in the cranial and spinal nerves. Influences from the cerebrum are projected to the lower brainstem reticular formation by (1) the corticoreticular fibers from the cerebral cortex and (2) the hypothalamotegmental, mamillotegmental, and dorsal longitudinal fasciculus from the hypothalamus and the limbic lobe. Other input to the brainstem reticular formation is derived from the spinal cord via the ascending spinoreticular fibers and from the cranial nerves. In turn, the influences from the brainstem reticular formation are conveyed via some of the reticulospinal fibers located in the anterior half of the spinal cord to the preganglionic neurons. These descending pathways are considered to be the upper motor neurons of the autonomic nervous system.

Interruption of the descending autonomic fibers in the brainstem or cervical spinal cord may result in Horner's syndrome (Chap. 10).

DENERVATION SENSITIVITY AND SYMPATHECTOMY

Some effectors are dependent upon their innervation for their structural and functional integrity. When denervated, they eventually become functionless and atrophy. This is the fate of denervated voluntary muscle as noted in a lower motor neuron paralysis (Chap. 10).

Other effectors are not wholly dependent upon their innervation to retain their functional status. Denervated involuntary muscles, cardiac muscles, and glands continue to function. For example, the transplanted heart may function adequately. However, when deprived of the autonomic nervous system influences, these effectors do not function absolutely normally in that they do not respond as effectively as they should to satisfy the changing demands of the organism.

When an effector is deprived of its innervation, it may become extremely sensitive to chemical mediators (neurotransmitters). For example, the rate of beat of the totally denervated heart will increase if the heart is exposed to but 1 part of epinephrine in 1,400 million. This *denervation hypersensitivity* is lost following the regeneration of the fibers and the reinnervation of the heart. Denervation hypersensitivity is noticeable in clinical situations following sympathectomy. In Horner's syndrome, the pupil of one eye is constricted and does not normally dilate, because it is deprived of sympathetic stimulation. However, when a patient with Horner's syndrome is extremely excited, the epinephrine and norepinephrine released by the adrenal medulla can stimulate the hypersensitive denervated dilator muscle of the iris to respond so that the pupil dilates; this is known as the *paradoxic pupillary response*.

ACTIVITY ON SPECIFIC ORGANS AND STRUCTURES

The response of a specific effector to a specific neurotransmitter is not solely determined by the neurotransmitter; the nature of the receptor sites on the effector is also significant in predicting the response to a stimulation. The response of an effector is determined by the nature of the neurotransmitter-receptor linkages. For example, norepinephrine stimulates the contraction of smooth muscles of an arteriole (vessel constricts) and the relaxation of smooth muscles of the bronchial tubes (tubes dilate) in the lungs. The different responses to the same neurosecretion are explained by the differences in the nature of the receptor sites on the smooth muscles. Different neurotransmitters may stimulate different effectors to respond in a similar way. For example, the radial muscle of the iris of the eye contracts when stimulated by norepinephrine, whereas the sphincter muscles of the iris contract when stimulated by acetylcholine; both are smooth muscles. (Refer to Table 17.1 to determine the response of various organs to sympathetic and parasympathetic stimulation.)

A dual innervation of the organs of the body by both the sympathetics and parasympathetics is general but not universal: (1) The heart has a true reciprocal (dual) innervation, with the sympathetics acting to increase and the parasympathetics acting to decrease the rate of the heartbeat. (2) The salivary glands are stimulated synergistically, with sympathetic activity producing a thick, viscous secretion and parasympathetic activity producing a profuse, watery secretion. (3) The constriction and dilatation of the pupil exemplifies an activity resulting from the stimulation of different muscle groups. The pupil of the eye dilates when the radial (dilator) muscles (innervated only by sympathetic fibers) are stimulated by the sympathetics, and it constricts when the sphincter (constrictor) muscles (innervated only by parasympathetic fibers) are stimulated by the parasympathetics. (4) Some structures are innervated by only one system; hair muscles (when goose pimples are formed) and sweat glands are stimulated only by sympathetic fibers.

ENTERIC NERVOUS SYSTEM

The neural networks and plexuses of the gastrointestinal canal should be considered as a distinct division of the autonomic nervous system called the enteric nervous system. The key feature of the enteric nervous system is its ability to carry on as a self-contained unit even when completely deprived of its innervation from the central nervous system.

The gastrointestinal tract contains intrinsic neural networks composed of sensory neurons, interneurons, and motor neurons. The motor neurons are actually the postganglionic parasympathetic neurons which receive neural influences from (1) the intrinsic sensory neurons and interneurons within the

Table 17.1   Some Comparisons between the Sympathetic and Parasympathetic Nervous Systems

General		
	Sympathetic nervous system	**Parasympathetic nervous system**
Outflow from CNS	Thoracolumbar levels	Craniosacral levels
Location of ganglia	Paravertebral and pre-vertebral ganglia close to CNS	Terminal ganglia near effectors
Ratio of preganglionic to postganglionic neurons	Each preganglionic neuron synapses with many postganglionic neurons	Each preganglionic neuron synapses with a few postganglionic neurons
Distribution in body	Throughout the body	Limited primarily to viscera of head, thorax, abdomen, and pelvis

Specific structures		
Structure	**Sympathetic function**	**Parasympathetic function**
Eye		
Radial muscle of iris	Dilates pupil (mydriasis)	
Sphincter muscle of iris		Contraction of pupil (miosis)
Ciliary muscle (accommodation)	Relaxation for far vision	Contraction for near vision
Glands of head		
Lacrimal gland		Stimulates secretion
Salivary glands	Scanty thick, viscous secretion	Profuse, watery secretion
Heart		
Rate	Increase	Decreased
Force of ventricular contraction	Increase	
Blood vessels	Generally constricts*	Slight effect
Lungs		
Bronchial tubes	Dilates lumen	Constricts lumen
Bronchial glands		Stimulates secretion
Gastrointestinal tract		
Motility and tone	Inhibits	Stimulates
Sphincters	Stimulates	Inhibits (relaxes)
Secretion	May inhibit	Stimulates
Gallbladder and ducts	Inhibits	Stimulates
Liver	Glycogenolysis increase (blood sugar)	

Table 17.1 *Continued*

Specific structures		
Structure	**Sympathetic function**	**Parasympathetic function**
Adrenal medulla	Secretion of epinephrine and norepinephrine*	
Sex organs	Vasoconstriction, constriction of vas deferens, seminal vesicle, and prostatic musculature (ejaculation)	Vasodilation and erection
Skin		
Sweat glands	Stimulated*	
Blood vessels	Constricted	Slight effect
Neurochemical basis		
	Sympathetic	**Parasympathetic**
Neurotransmitter at neuro-effector junction	Usually norepinephrine*	Acetylcholine
Inactivation of transmitter	Slow and reuptake	Rapid
Reinforcement in body	Secretion of norepinephrine and epinephrine by adrenal medulla	

* Exceptions: Some postganglionic neurons of the sympathetic nervous system are cholinergic neurons. Sympathetic neuroeffector transmission mediated by acetylcholine includes (1) some blood vessels in skeletal muscles and (2) most sweat glands. The sweat glands of the palms are innervated by adrenergic fibers. The adrenal medulla is innervated by preganglionic cholinergic sympathetic neurons.

gut and (2) the preganglionic parasympathetic neurons. The *intrinsic sensory neurons* with cell bodies located within the submucosa receive input from their dendritic processes in the mucosa; these neurons have axons which interact with the interneurons and postganglionic neurons of the submucosal (Meissner's) plexus and the myenteric (Auerbach's) plexus. This intrinsic neural network is an integrating complex exerting excitatory and inhibitory influences on the smooth muscle of the muscularis mucosa and the external muscular lamina.

The sensory neurons can initiate a coordinated *peristaltic reflex* in the intestinal tract. This neuronal network comprises the components of an intrinsic reflex pathway. In the "law of the intestine," stimulation of the gut causes contraction above the point of stimulus and relaxation below. This peristaltic reflex is elicited by moderate distention. Inhibition of intestinal tone and motility produced by distention of some other part of the gut is called the *intestino-intestinal inhibitory reflex*. In addition, the visceral myogenic smooth muscle activity is modulated by extrinsic excitatory motor (parasympathetic) and inhibitory (sympathetic) fibers.

Chapter 18

Hypothalamus

The 4-g hypothalamus is located in the basal region of the diencephalon adjacent to the third ventricle. In its rostrocaudal extent from the lamina terminalis to the midbrain, the hypothalamus is divided into nuclei and four major areas (Figs. 18.1 and 18.2): (1) a rostral or preoptic area, (2) a supraoptic area located above the optic chiasma, (3) a tuberal area (the region of tuber cinereum extends from optic chiasm to mamillary body), and (4) a caudal or mamillary area which grades into the midbrain central gray. The *hypophysis* (pituitary gland) extends ventrally from the tuberal area. Some important hypothalamic nuclei include the paraventricular nucleus and supraoptic nucleus of the supraoptic area, the lateral and ventral medial nuclei of the tuberal area, and the mamillary nuclei of the mamillary area (Figs. 18.1 and 18.2).

The hypophysis (pituitary gland) comprises two major subdivisions—the *adenohypophysis* (an epithelial structure) and the *neurohypophysis* (a neural structure). The adenohypophysis develops as an outpocketing from the embryonic pharynx, while the neurohypophysis originates as an outgrowth from the region of neural tube giving rise to the hypothalamus. The adenohy-

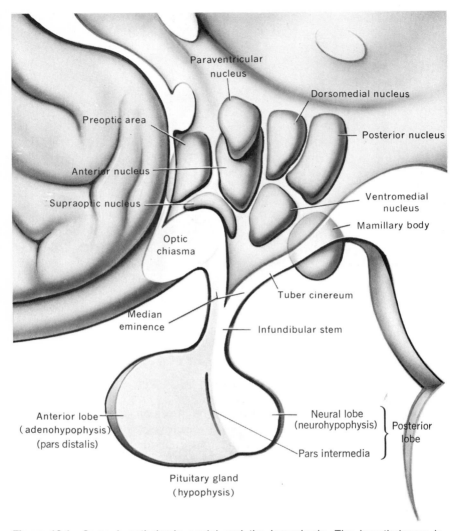

Figure 18.1 Some hypothalamic nuclei and the hypophysis. The hypothalamus is composed of four nuclear areas: (1) nuclei of the preoptic area (telencephalic region); (2) nuclei of the supraoptic or anterior area, including the paraventricular nucleus, anterior nucleus, and supraoptic nucleus; (3) nuclei of the tuberal or middle area, including the dorsomedial and ventromedial nuclei; and (4) nuclei of the mamillary or posterior area, including the posterior nucleus and the mamillary body.

pophysis consists of the pars distalis (anterior lobe), pars tuberalis, and pars intermedia (Fig. 18.1). The neurohypophysis comprises the median eminence of the tuber cinereum, infundibular stem, and infundibular process (pars nervosa, neural lobe, Fig. 18.2). The median eminence, which extends from the optic chiasm to the infundibular stem, differs from the rest of the hypothalamus. The median eminence and the infundibular stem are known as the *hypophysiotropic area,* where the neurally derived hypothalamic releasing hormones are released and transferred to the hypophysial portal system.

GENERAL FUNCTIONAL CONSIDERATIONS

The hypothalamus exerts significant roles in numerous visceromotor and behavioral responses through the autonomic nervous system, endocrine system, and even through the somatic motor system. It functions primarily in *homeostasis*—the maintenance of a relatively constant internal body environment (e.g., constant body temperature) through the activities of regulatory centers and modulating centers.

A *regulatory (integration) center* is a crucial control center which is essential to the expression of a specific function; an example is the "thermostat" monitoring and controlling body temperature, located in the hypothalamus. A *modulating center* is a nuclear pool influencing a regulation center. It is not vital to a specific function. The hypothalamus can influence the blood

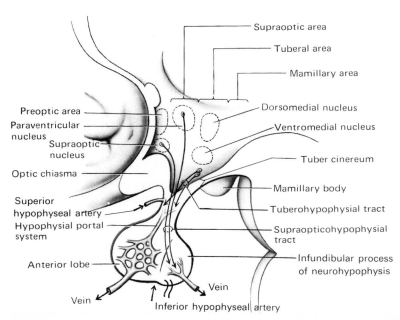

Figure 18.2 Some hypothalamic nuclei and the hypophysis. The supraopticohypophyseal tract extends from the supraoptic and paraventricular nucleus to the capillary bed of the neurohypophysis. The hypophyseal-portal system is a vascular network extending from the base of the hypothalamus and upper neurohypophysis to the anterior lobe of the hypophysis.

pressure regulatory (integration) centers in the medulla. Through these roles the hypothalamus exerts influences upon behavioral responses in both visceromotor and somatomotor spheres.

Intrinsic Hypothalamic Receptors

Some neurons within the hypothalamus act as intrinsic receptors involved in several vital functional activities—thermal receptors for temperature regulation and osmoreceptors for water metabolism. For example, to perform its role as the integrator of body temperature, the hypothalamic receptors monitor the temperature of the blood flowing through the hypothalamic capillaries. The efferent arms of this receptor include (1) descending autonomic pathways to the sweat glands and peripheral blood vessels and (2) descending somatic pathways to the trunk musculature (panting and shivering).

Neurohumoral Reflexes

This arc utilizes both the nervous system (neuro-) and the blood vascular system (humoral). To perform its role in water metabolism, for example, the hypothalamus utilizes an intrinsic hypothalamic receptor to monitor the osmolality of the blood flowing through the brain. The neuron receptors are stimulated to release a neurosecretion, antidiuretic hormone (ADH), which is conveyed via nerve fibers (*supraopticohypophysial tract*) to the infundibular process of the hypophysis (Fig. 18.2), where it is stored and released into the systemic blood system and conveyed to its target structures in the kidney. Such reflexes are discussed more fully below.

Hypophysial Portal System and Hypothalamic Releasing Hormones

The hypophysis receives its blood supply from several arteries (Fig. 18.2). A pair of inferior hypophysial arteries from the internal carotid arteries furnish blood to the infundibular process and infundibular stem. Several superior hypophysial arteries from the internal carotid arteries form a capillary plexus in the median eminence, pars tuberalis, and infundibular stem; this capillary plexus collects into the *hypophysial portal system* of blood vessels (hypothalamic portal system and hypophysial portal vein). This portal system is a vascular network commencing as a capillary bed in the median eminence and collecting into several main channels before arborizing into a capillary (sinusoidal) bed in the adenohypophysis (Fig. 18.2).

The hypophysial portal system is the vascular pathway through which the neural language from the hypophysiotropic area, in the form of releasing hormones (RH), is transferred and conveyed to the pars anterior to trigger the endocrine language of the hypophysis. More specifically, the hypothalamic nerve fibers liberate the releasing hormones from these nerve endings into the capillary plexuses of the median eminence and infundibular stem; these hormones are conveyed through the hypophysial portal vessels to the adenohypophysis, where they stimulate or inhibit the release of a number of the hypophysial hormones. The *hypothalamic hormones* known to control the release of hypophysial hormones include corticotropin RH, thyrotropin RH, luteinizing hormone RH, follicle-stimulating hormone RH, growth hormone RH, prolactin RH, and melanocyte-stimulating hormone RH. Other hormones include the growth hormone (release)-inhibiting hormone, prolactin (release)-inhibiting hormone, and melanocyte-stimulating and (release)-inhibiting hormones.

BASIC CIRCUITS OF THE HYPOTHALAMUS

The hypothalamus is strategically located between the cerebrum and the brainstem. The complex neural circuits associated with the hypothalamus have reciprocal and widespread connections with these regions (Figs. 19.2 and 19.3). The hypothalamus derives its major input from the nonspecific reticular pathways and little, if any, from the specific lemniscal pathways. The structures projecting to and receiving from the hypothalamus include the brainstem reticular formation, limbic lobe (including hippocampus and amygdaloid body), thalamus, and olfactory pathways. The major pathway of the hypothalamus is the medial forebrain bundle. This is an intricate complex of short, multisynaptic, multineuronal chains extending from parts of the limbic lobe through the lateral hypothalamus to the paramedian tegmentum of the midbrain.

Input (Fig. 18.3)

The *input to the hypothalamus* is conveyed via (1) ascending pathways from the brainstem tegmentum and periaqueductal gray matter, (2) descending fibers from the forebrain, and (3) the blood vascular system.

1   The *ascending pathways from the brainstem* include fibers of the mamillary peduncle from the dorsal and ventral tegmental nuclei, fibers of the dorsal longitudinal fasciculus from the periaqueductal gray matter, fibers of the medial forebrain bundle from the midbrain tegmentum, and catecholamine pathways from some brainstem nuclei (Chap. 11 and Figs. 11.6 and 21.4).
2   The *descending fibers from the forebrain* include (Fig. 18.3):
a   Fibers of the fornix originating in the hippocampus and the septal nuclei of the limbic system. The hippocampus is a significant channel for afferent and neocortical input to the hypothalamus.
b   Fibers originating in cortex of the uncus and amygdaloid body. These project via the stria terminalis and ventral amygdalofugal pathway to the hypothalamus. The primary olfactory cortex project via fibers of the

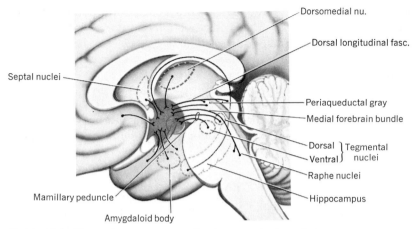

Dorsomedial nu.

Dorsal longitudinal fasc.

Septal nuclei

Periaqueductal gray

Medial forebrain bundle

Dorsal ⎫ Tegmental
Ventral ⎭   nuclei

Raphe nuclei

Mamillary peduncle

Hippocampus

Amygdaloid body

Figure 18.3 The major tracts conveying input to the hypothalamus.

medial forebrain bundle. The olfactory system is the only sensory system with a direct route to the hypothalamus. A few fibers from the retina terminate in the hypothalamus (suprachiasmatic nucleus).

c The orbitofrontal cortex and septal nuclei, the source of fibers of the medial forebrain bundle.

d The dorsomedial and midline nuclei of the thalamus which project to the hypothalamus and amygdaloid body.

3 The *blood vascular system* conveys influences to which the hypothalamus may respond. These include hormones, temperature of the blood, and osmolality of the blood plasma.

Output (Fig. 18.4)

The *output from the hypothalamus* is conveyed via (1) ascending fibers to the forebrain, (2) descending fibers to the midbrain and pons, and (3) fibers and blood vessels to the hypophysis (endocrine effector projections).

1 The *ascending fibers from the hypothalamus to the forebrain* include those projecting to the anterior and dorsomedial thalamic nuclei, septal nuclei, and septal (subcallosal) area.

2 The *descending fibers* to the midbrain and pons project to the dorsal and ventral tegmental nuclei, superior central nucleus (a raphe nucleus), and the periaqueductal gray matter. The descending tracts from the hypothalamus include the dorsal longitudinal fasciculus, medial forebrain bundle, and mamillotegmental fasciculus.

3 The influences from the *hypothalamus to the hypophysis* are conveyed via the hypophysial portal system to the adenohypophysis and via the supraopticohypophysial tract to the neural lobe (see below).

These projections to and from the hypothalamus are involved with the functional activities of the autonomic nervous system (Chap. 17), limbic system (Chap. 19), and endocrine system (see below).

NEUROHUMORAL REFLEXES

The hypothalamus is integrated into distinct neurohumoral reflexes, in which two separate fiber pathways extend from the hypothalamus to the hypophysis. The neurons of these pathways are involved with both neurally and humorally conveyed stimuli.

Tuberohypophysial Tract

The tuberohypophysial tract projects from the hypothalamic nuclei in the tuber cinereum and terminates in the infundibular stem. The neurons of this tract elaborate and convey the hypophysial hormone–releasing hormones (hypophysiotropic hormones, hypothalamic releasing factors) to the capillary loops of the hypophysial portal system and via this system to the adenohypophysis, where releasing hormones trigger the emission of various hypophysial hormones into the systemic bloodstream. There is probably a different releasing hormone for each of the hypophysial tropic hormones.

The hypophysial tropic hormones include (1) corticotropin (adrenocorticotropic hormone, ACTH), which regulates the growth and secretion of the cortex of the adrenal gland, (2) thyrotropic hormone, which has similar actions on the thyroid gland, (3) follicle-stimulating hormone (FSH), which is involved in the growth and maturation of ovarian follicles up

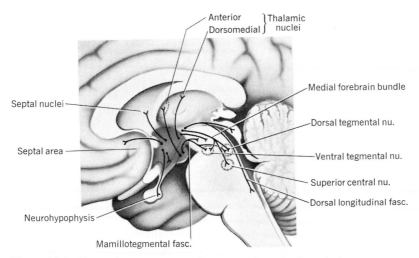

Figure 18.4 The major tracts conveying output from the hypothalamus.

to the time of ovulation, (4) luteinizing hormone (LH), which, acting together with FSH, induces ovulation and then stimulates the formation and secretion of the corpus luteum, (5) growth (somatotropic) hormone, which regulates somatic growth and influences metabolism, (6) prolactin (lactotropin, lactogenic hormone), which is involved with the secretion of milk after the mammary gland has developed in response to ovarian hormones FSH and LH, and (7) melanocyte-stimulating hormone of the pars intermedia, which in mammals appears to have an effect on melanin pigment formation.

These are also hypothalamic pituitary hormone–inhibiting hormones: growth hormone (release)–inhibiting hormone, prolactin (release)–inhibiting hormone, and melanocyte (release)–inhibiting hormone.

A complex series of several *feedback systems* have a significant role in regulating and controlling the secretory activity of these hormones. They comprise (1) a *long feedback loop,* in which the hypothalamus monitors hormones synthesized by the peripheral target organs (e.g., thyroxin released by the thyroid gland is fed back via the bloodstream to be monitored by the hypothalamus), (2) a *short feedback loop,* in which each tropic hormone of the pituitary gland is fed back to and monitored by the hypothalamus, (3) an even *shorter feedback loop,* in which the releasing hormones feed back to and are monitored by the hypothalamus, and (4) a *feedback loop* in which each tropic hormone within the tissues is fed back to the hypophysis to influence and to regulate the release of the same tropic hormone (e.g., growth hormone).

Supraopticohypophysial Tract

The *supraopticohypophysial tract* (Fig. 18.2), made up of about 100,000 unmyelinated fibers, extends from the supraoptic and paraventricular nuclei to the capillary bed of the neurohypophysis (posterior lobe). The fibers convey, via axoplasmatic transport, *antidiuretic hormone* (ADH, vasopressin), which is involved with the homeostatic role of conserving water, and *oxytocin,* which has a role in stimulating the contraction of smooth muscles of the uterus and of myoepithelial cells of the mammary glands. These hormones are released into the systemic circulation within the capillaries of the neurohypophysis.

AUTONOMIC NERVOUS SYSTEM

The hypothalamus is the chief *subcortical* center regulating all kinds of visceral activities and some somatic functions; it acts primarily as a modulator of autonomic centers in the brainstem and spinal cord (Chap. 17).

The *anterior hypothalamus* (preoptic and supraoptic regions) has an excitatory parasympathetic (or inhibitory to sympathetic activity) role. The stimulation of this region may produce a decrease in the rate of the heartbeat, decrease in blood pressure, dilatation of the cutaneous blood vessels, increase in motility, peristalsis, and secretion in the gastrointestinal tract, constriction of the pupil, and increased sweating. Activity in this region produces a parasympathetic (vagal) tone and such somatic responses as panting. Lesions in this area may result in the production of sympathetic effects.

The *posterior hypothalamus* has an excitatory sympathetic role. Activation of this region may produce an increase in the rate of the heartbeat, increase in blood pressure, constriction of cutaneous blood vessels, decrease in motility, peristalsis, and secretion in the gastrointestinal tract, dilatation of the pupil, and erection of hair. Activity in this region produces a sympathetic tone and such somatic responses as shivering, running, and struggling.

TEMPERATURE REGULATION

The hypothalamus has an essential role in body temperature: it regulates the balance between heat production and heat loss. More specifically, the hypothalamus has thermal receptor neurons which monitor the temperature of the blood. This "thermostat" regulates the heat-producing and heat-conserving control systems. In effect, the continuous fine adjustments necessary for maintaining a constant normal body temperature depend upon the hypothalamus.

The anterior hypothalamus acts to prevent a rise in body temperature. It activates those processes which favor heat loss including vasodilatation of cutaneous blood vessels, sweating (evaporation of water for cooling), and panting. Destruction of this "heat-dissipating region" may produce a highly elevated body temperature (hyperthermia).

The posterior hypothalamus contains a region which triggers those activities concerned with heat production and heat conservation. These include the metabolic heat-producing systems (oxidation of glucose), vasoconstriction (especially of cutaneous blood vessels), erection of hair (goose pimples), and shivering. The malfunctioning of this region may produce a cold-blooded (poikilothermic) mammal that cannot sustain a uniform body temperature.

Pyrogenic substances, produced in some diseases, affect the hypothalamus. A fever known as *neurogenic hyperthermia* results.

REGULATION OF WATER BALANCE

The hypothalamus has significant roles in fluid balance by regulating both the intake (by drinking) and output (through kidneys and sweat glands) of water. Evidence indicates that a "drinking" or "thirst" center is located in the lateral hypothalamus and a "thirst satiety" center in the medial hypothalamus. The *osmoreceptor neurons* in these hypothalamic centers respond to the osmolality of the blood passing through these nuclei. They set off events which stimulate or inhibit water intake. Other factors such as dryness of the oral mucosa from decreased salivary flow also influence intake of water.

The hypothalamus has a crucial role in the conservation and loss of body water through the regulation of urine flow in the kidneys by ADH, which is produced by the neurons of the supraoptic and paraventricular nuclei of the hypothalamus. ADH (vasopressin) is synthesized by the neurons in these nuclei and carried by axoplasmatic transport in the supraoptico-hypophysial tract to the neurohypophysis (Fig. 18.2), where it is stored or released into the systemic blood circulation. The ADH acts upon the kidney (distal convoluted and collecting tubules) to increase the reabsorption of water from the dilute glomerular filtrate in the tubules back into the blood-stream, thus concentrating the urine. Water is thereby conserved and is not excreted in the urine. Increases in osmolality in blood flowing through the hypothalamus stimulate the release of ADH; this results in antidiuresis and conservation of water. Decreases in osmolality inhibit the release of ADH; this results in diuresis and excretion of water in urine. Other factors may have a role; vascular receptors monitoring blood volume or flow in the body project input to the hypothalamus, in this way influencing the release of ADH.

A deficiency in the formation and release of ADH may result in *diabetes insipidus* (increased excretion of water without increase in sugar), in which as much as 15 to 25 gal of urine may be excreted per day.

FOOD INTAKE AND ENERGY BALANCE

The hypothalamic region involved with feeding responses has been called the "appestat," with the ventral medial hypothalamic nucleus called the "satiety center" and the lateral hypothalamic nucleus called the "hunger" or "feed-ing" center. Stimulation of the ventral median nucleus inhibits the animal's urge to eat. Destruction of this nucleus produces an animal exhibiting decreased physical activity and a voracious appetite (not true hunger) with a twofold to threefold increase in food intake. The animal becomes obese. Stimulation of the lateral hypothalamic nucleus induces the animal to eat, whereas its destruction produces an animal that refuses to eat until severe emaciation from starvation ensues.

Two theories have been proposed to explain how these centers are influenced. According to the *glucostat hypothesis,* hypothalamic neurons respond to the blood glucose levels. According to the *thermostat hypothesis,* blood temperature is the causative factor, with an increase resulting from the specific dynamic action of ingested food and with a decrease resulting from dissipation of heat through the skin.

EXPRESSIONS OF EMOTION AND BEHAVIOR

The behavioral patterns associated with emotional experiences are of two general types: (1) subjective "feelings" and (2) objective physical expressions. The subjective aspects of emotion, from depression to euphoria, are more intimately bound up with the cerebral cortex. Many of the objective physical expressions are largely mediated through the hypothalamus and are recognizable as the enhanced activity of the autonomic nervous system. They include alterations in the heartbeat (palpitations) and the blood pressure, blushing and pallor of the face, dryness of the mouth, clammy hands, dilatation of the pupil (glassy eye), cold sweat, tears of happiness or sadness, and changes in the concentration of the blood sugar. Stimulation of the hypothalamus in man is said to evoke changes in the blood pressure and the rate of the heartbeat without any psychic manifestations.

"Pleasure Centers" and "Punishing Centers" (See Chap. 19)
Sleep-Wake Cycle

The hypothalamus is associated with the state of awakeness and integrated somehow into the sleep-wake cycle. The *ascending reticular activating system* (*ARAS*), which projects to the hypothalamus, and the diffuse projections from the hypothalamus to the cerebral cortex are among the neural substrates for the sleep-wake cycle (Chap. 19). The bilateral ablation of the regions posterolateral and caudal to the mamillary bodies produces a tame, apathetic, and often somnolent monkey or cat. Stimulation of the hypothalamus may induce drowsiness and sleep.

Chapter 19

Reticular System and Limbic System

The *reticular system* and the *limbic system* are physiologic systems which are described in terms of functional criteria that vary from definite to difficult-to-define. The structural matrices utilized by these systems include some imprecisely delineated neuroanatomic pathways, "networks," and nuclear complexes. These systems are most useful as concepts relating to a number of functional expressions of the nervous system. Authorities differ in their interpretations and evaluations of the structural and functional aspects of these systems.

RETICULAR SYSTEM

The *reticular system* has a role in consciousness and the associated states grading from sleep, drowsiness, and relaxation through alertness and attention—otherwise known as the sleep-wake cycle. These states are expressed in the electroencephalogram (EEG). In addition, this system is involved, mainly in the background, in the perception and discrimination of sensory input and in the modification of behavior. The ascending influences are processed and conveyed via the ascending reticular system (ARS), and the descending influences projected by descending somatic pathways (primarily corticoreticulospinal pathway) and the autonomic nervous system. The system involved with the sleep-wake cycle is referred to as the ascending reticular activating system (ARAS).

LIMBIC SYSTEM

The *limbic system* is recognized as the mediator of those vague and variegated qualities known as the affective or feeling state or mood and instinct. It is involved with emotional behavior as expressed through endocrine, visceral, and somatic activities. This system is integral to those actions essential to the self-preservation of the organism, e.g., feeding, fight, and fright, and to the preservation of the species, e.g., mating, procreation, and care of offspring. The main outlets for limbic system activity are (1) pathways from the hypothalamus and midbrain tegmentum (central focal sites for discharge) to the brainstem and spinal cord (via autonomic nervous system, descending reticular pathways, and somatic nervous system), and (2) the pathways to the hypophysis and the endocrine system.

The *anatomic substrates of the limbic system* are located in the limbic lobe, some subcortical nuclei, such as the septal nuclei and the amygdaloid body, and neural pathways to other nuclear stations of the brain (Figs. 19.1 to 19.3). The "other" nuclei include the habenular nucleus, hypothalamus, medial midbrain tegmentum, parts of the thalamus, and the interpeduncular nucleus of the midbrain. The *limbic lobe* comprises portions of the subcallosal area, cingulate gyrus, isthmus, parahippocampal gyrus, hippocampal formation, dentate gyrus, and uncus (primary olfactory cortex, Fig. 1.3). The cortex of the limbic lobe is phylogenetically old cortex called the *archicortex* and *paleocortex* (collectively called *allocortex*). The *septal region* includes septal nuclei in the septum pellucidum and cortex rostral to the anterior commissure.

ANATOMY OF THE RETICULAR SYSTEM

The anatomic substrate for the reticular system is the core reticular pathway found throughout the neuraxis of the central nervous system. In man and the other mammals, it represents the evolved product of the pathways with an ancient phylogenetic history. The well-organized pathway is conceived of as located throughout the neuraxis from spinal cord through cerebral cortex (Fig. 19.1). The pathway is presumed to consist of neurons and tracts within the following structures: (1) cells in laminae V, VI, VII, and VIII of the spinal cord and the ascending spinoreticular and descending reticulospinal tracts, (2) reticular nuclei of the massive reticular formation of the brainstem

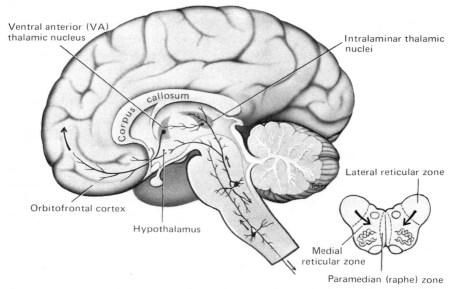

Figure 19.1 Schematic representation of the ascending projections of the ascending reticular pathway system. In general, the multineuronal, multisynaptic relays of the brainstem reticular formation (located in the tegmentum) extend rostrally into two telencephalic regions: (1) posteriorly into the intralaminar, ventral anterior (VA), and dorsomedial thalamic nuclear complexes, and (2) anteriorly into the hypothalamus. The thalamic component projects, via the VA thalamic nucleus, to the orbitofrontal cortex.

The cross section through the brainstem (medulla) illustrates the division of the brainstem reticular formation into a midline raphe or paramedian zone, a medial reticular or "motor" zone, and a lateral reticular or "sensory" zone. Arrows indicate the general direction of flow of neural influences.

tegmentum and its central tegmental tract (both ascending and descending projections), (3) a posterior extension ascending rostrally to the intralaminar and ventral anterior thalamic nuclei and then to the fronto-orbital cortex, and (4) an anterior extension ascending through the subthalamus and hypothalamus and then, possibly, to the limbic cortex. Descending influences from the cerebrum are probably conveyed via corticoreticular fibers, medial forebrain bundle, and thalamotegmental fibers (collaterals from intralaminar nuclei to midbrain tegmentum).

The *brainstem reticular formation* (*central brainstem core*) is subdivided at all levels into three zones (Fig. 19.1): (1) nuclei of the *midline raphe and paramedian zone,* (2) nuclei of the *medial zone* (comprises the medial two-thirds of the tegmentum with such nuclei as the nucleus reticularis giganto-cellularis of the medulla and nuclei reticularis pontis caudalis and oralis of the pons), and (3) nuclei of the lateral zone (comprises the lateral one-third). The *lateral reticular zone* ("sensory zone," see Chap. 11) is composed of small cells with relatively short ascending and descending axons which terminate primarily medially in the medial reticular zone. This zone is considered to be an afferent and association area because it receives multiple "sensory" input from the spinal cord, cranial nerves, and cerebrum. The *medial reticular zone* ("motor zone," see Chap. 11) consists of many large cells with numerous long axons, each of which bifurcates in a long ascending and a long descending fiber; these fibers form the *central tegmental tract* of the brainstem tegmentum. Many of the ascending fibers (both crossed and uncrossed) from the medulla and lower pons extend rostrally to the midbrain, the hypothalamus, and intralaminar thalamic nuclei (Fig. 19.1). Descending fibers project via the medial and lateral reticulospinal tracts to the spinal cord (Fig. 9.2).

In general, the brainstem reticular formation is not diffuse but well organized in an orderly and precise manner, with (1) the dendrites of each "reticular" neuron oriented in the transverse plane at right angles to the neuraxis of the brainstem, and (2) the ascending and descending branches of the bifurcated axon oriented parallel to the long axis of the brainstem (Fig. 19.1). Numerous collateral branches leave the main axonic branches. This organization permits a tremendous amount of neuronal interaction. The overlap of axonal branches suggests that specificity of input cannot always be maintained; with the convergence of somatosensory, acoustic, and vestibular impulses on the same neuronal units, modality specificity is lost or modified. The basic input to the brainstem reticular formation is derived from the spinal cord via spinoreticular fibers and collaterals of ascending pathways

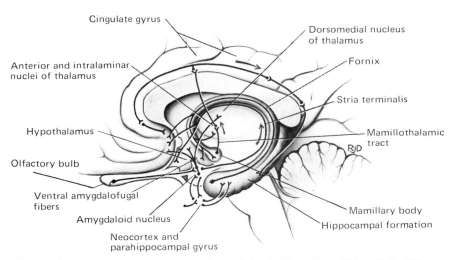

Figure 19.2 Schema of some connections of the limbic system. Note (A) the "Papez circuit" composed of hippocampal formation, fornix, mamillary body, anterior nucleus of thalamus, and cingulate cortex, and (B) amygdaloid nucleus and its connections. James W. Papez proposed circuit A in 1937.

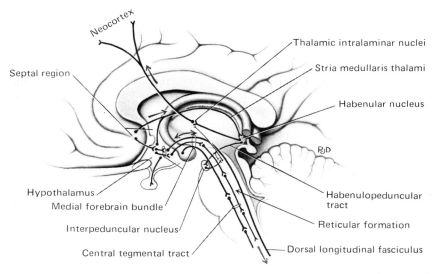

Neocortex

Septal region

Thalamic intralaminar nuclei

Stria medullaris thalami

Habenular nucleus

$R_{J}D$

Hypothalamus

Medial forebrain bundle

Interpeduncular nucleus

Central tegmental tract

Habenulopeduncular tract

Reticular formation

Dorsal longitudinal fasciculus

Figure 19.3 Schema of some connections of the limbic system. Note (A) the medial forebrain bundle which extends from the septal region through the lateral hypothalamus to the midbrain reticular formation, and (B) the sequence of septal region, habenular nucleus, interpeduncular nucleus, and midbrain reticular formation.

from collateral branches of all cranial nerves (especially ns. V, VIII, IX, and X), from the cerebellum, and from the cerebrum (hypothalamus, basal ganglia, limbic lobe, and neocortex) via hypothalamotegmental, pallidotegmental, and corticoreticular fibers. The basic output from the brainstem reticular formation is directed (1) caudally via the reticulospinal tracts to the spinal cord (Fig. 9.2), (2) laterally to the cranial nerve nuclei, (3) rostrally via the central tegmental tract to the hypothalamus, septal region, and the midline and intralaminar thalamic nuclei, and (4) to the cerebellum. The monoamine pathways are integrated into the ascending projections (Chaps. 11 and 21; Figs. 11.6 and 21.4). One aspect of the rostral projection involves the pathway by which influences are conveyed by the intralaminar thalamic nuclei [and part of the ventral anterior (VA) thalamic nucleus] to the cerebral cortex. Appropriate stimulation of these nuclei produces physiologic events over the entire cortex; yet projections from these nuclei to the entire cortex are not readily demonstrable anatomically. Recent evidence suggests that neurons of the intralaminar nuclei have, in addition to their direct and abundant projections to the striatum (Chap. 21), diffuse and sparse collateral projections to the cerebral cortex. These collateral fibers along with the relatively dense projections from VA to the orbitofrontal cortex may be the morphological substrate for some of the functional activity noted below.

FUNCTION OF THE RETICULAR SYSTEM

The reticular system is an integrating system in which influences from the sensory modalities as well as from cerebral, cerebellar, and spinal and cranial nerve sources converge and interact. The neural networks of the reticular system convey and process these influences which become associated with vaguely appreciated senses, such as poorly localized pain, neural activities associated with the sleep-wake cycle, and affective behavioral expressions.

The ARAS has roles in the alteration of states of consciousness and attention and in the modification of the reception, conduction, perception, and discrimination of sensory input. The ascending reticular pathways, acting potently through the intralaminar and VA thalamic nuclei and intra-thalamic connections with other thalamic nuclei (see Chap. 20), influence the activity of the cerebral cortex; this ARAS may result in either (1) widespread electrocortical synchronization and behavioral sleep, or (2) widespread electrocortical desynchronization and arousal following appropriate stimulation. In response to stimulation (even an external stimulus), there is a parallelism between the state of consciousness and the record of the EEG. When the human subject is in a state of relaxation or drowsiness, the EEG is said to exhibit a *synchronized pattern*, on the assumption that many cortical neurons are in synchronous activity. The brain waves have a high-voltage, slow-frequency rhythm (HVS) of 50 μV at a frequency of 8 to 14 per second. The *"deactivated" pattern* (*alpha rhythm*) is most prominent in the occipital region when the eyes are closed. When the subject passes from relaxation to an alert, attentive state, the resting alpha rhythm is replaced by an irregular, reduced-amplitude, rapid oscillation (desynchronization of alpha rhythm or alpha blocking) called the *beta* pattern. It is present during states of attention and problem solving. This activated or arousal rhythm is a low-voltage, fast-frequency rhythm (LVF) of 5 to 10 μV at a frequency of from 15 to 30 per second. This "desynchronized" EEG or "activation" pattern is most prominent in the frontal and parietal regions. When the subject passes from the wakeful state to sleep, the desynchronized (LVF) activity in the cerebral cortex gradually shifts to the synchronized (HVS) rhythm with so-called "spindle bursts."

Different stimuli exert their influences differentially upon the ARAS. Acoustic stimuli are more effective than visual stimuli. Pain conveyed via the trigeminal nerve and spinal nerves has fairly potent effects upon evoking desynchronization (arousal). The general anesthetics, including pentobarbital and volatile anesthetics, tend to block transmission through the ARAS but do not affect the specific lemniscal pathways. The latter continue to convey their influences. The ARAS activity is increased by such humorally conveyed agents as epinephrine and carbon dioxide.

Lesions of the midbrain and diencephalon may result in loss of con-

sciousness (*coma*), which may last for months, accompanied by synchronization (HVS) of EEG, slow respiration, and muscular relaxation. This is
presumably due to injury to the reticular formation; the upper brainstem is
apparently essential for "crude consciousness." The complex interactions
within the reticular system may, through fluctuations of their responsiveness
to "sensory" stimuli, produce a variability in their effect upon the nuances of
sleep, drowsiness, attentiveness, and alertness.

The reticular system also exerts its influences on visceral activities (e.g.,
heartbeat and digestive system) and on phasic and tonic motor activities (e.g.,
fidgeting and relaxation).

ANATOMY OF THE LIMBIC SYSTEM

The following outline describes the more salient interconnections and circuits
(many are reciprocal) of the limbic system (Figs. 19.2 and 19.3). The precise
functional significance of each of these possible circuits is not resolved.

Circuits: (1) The cells in the hippocampus have axons extending
through the fornix and terminating in the anterior and intralaminar nuclei of
the thalamus, septal area, septal nuclei, and hypothalamus, especially the
mamillary body. Cells in the mamillary body project axons via the mamillothalamic tract to the anterior nucleus of the thalamus, which, in turn, projects
fibers to the cingulate gyrus of the limbic lobe. From this gyrus a multineuronal pathway terminates in the hippocampus to complete the circuit.
The hippocampus receives input from the neocortex and paleocortex. (2)
Fibers from the amygdaloid body project to the subcallosal area (cortex just
rostral to lamina terminalis, septal nuclei (nuclei in vicinity of anterior
commissure and septum pellucidum), hypothalamus, and dorsomedial nucleus of the thalamus. These projections from the amygdaloid body are via
both the stria terminalis (parallels fornix) and the ventral amygdalofugal
projection. Inputs to the corticomedial nuclear group of the amygdaloid body
are derived from the olfactory system, and those to the basolateral nuclear
group of the amygdaloid body are derived from the neocortex. In brief, the
amygdaloid body receives its major input from the olfactory system and
projects its major output to the septal area and hypothalamus. (3) The
multineuronal pathway composed of cells with short axons extends from the
subcallosal area through the lateral hypothalamus to the medial midbrain
tegmentum. This medial forebrain bundle has reciprocal connections. (4)
Fibers from the subcallosal area, septal region, and anterior hypothalamus
pass via the stria medullaris thalami to the habenular nucleus and from this
nucleus via the habenulopeduncular tract to the midbrain (interpeduncular
nucleus and medial midbrain tegmentum). (5) The amygdaloid body projects
directly and topographically to the prefrontal lobe (cortex).

These circuits have connections with the opposite side via anterior commissure and hippocampal commissure. Many influences are relayed to these circuits. Note that these circuits are integrated into other functional systems: (1) midbrain tegmentum and medial forebrain bundle with the reticular system and the hypothalamus, (2) dorsomedial nucleus of thalamus with the prefrontal cortex (Chap. 22), and (3) intralaminar nuclei of the thalamus with the reticular system.

FUNCTION OF THE LIMBIC SYSTEM

The structures associated with the limbic lobe and limbic system are somehow involved with matters related to feeling states and behavior.

Stimulation of Structures within the Limbic System

Electric stimulation of the amygdaloid body and immediate region in the unanesthetized monkey produces a number of behavioral actions. Activities associated with feeding and nutrition are elicited, including sniffing, licking, biting, swallowing, and retching movements. Monkeys exhibit *agonistic behavior patterns*—behavior manifested by animals in an attack-and-defense contest during fight or fright. The peaceful monkey becomes a furious and aggressive animal that attacks and bullies; once the stimulus is turned off, the peaceful monkey reappears. The increase in the secretion of digestive juices in the alimentary canal after repeated acute stimulations of the amygdaloid body may be followed by the appearance of gastric erosions similar to peptic ulcers in the stomachs of monkeys. The possibility of psychic factors in the production of peptic ulcers in man is implied.

Stimulation of the hippocampal formation may result in respiratory and cardiovascular changes and in a generalized arousal response. In the expression of arousal the formation acts as a supplemental motor area by inducing such somatic movements as facial grimaces, shoulder shrugging, and hand movements, which are considered to be normal behavioral gestures.

Responses indicative of activity of the autonomic nervous system are evoked by stimulation of the cingulate gyrus and septal area. Some responses, even observed in man, include changes in the tone of the blood vascular system, in respiratory rhythms, and in the activity of the digestive system.

Aggressiveness can be inhibited or decreased in monkeys by stimulating the septal area. The stimulation of the septal area of the "boss" monkey with implanted electrodes reduces the aggressive behavior of this dominant monkey. If stimulation is prolonged over a period of days, the other monkeys of the colony sense this change. They lose their fear of the "boss" and take new liberties, such as invading his territory and securing a larger share of food. The former situation returns after stimulations cease.

"Pleasure Centers" and "Punishing Centers"

The stimulation by implanted electrodes of certain regions of the limbic system drives the animal to seek further stimulation. The animal will trip the lever over and over again and thus continually restimulate itself—an expression of positive reinforcement on self-stimulation. Such nodal sites have been named "pleasure centers" or "rewarding centers." The stimulation of some regions excites the animal to avoid further stimulation—an expression of negative reinforcement on self-stimulation. Such sites have been named "punishing centers" or "aversion centers." The so-called pleasure centers have been located in the subcallosal area, cingulate cortex, hippocampal formation, amygdaloid body, hypothalamus, midbrain tegmentum, and anterior nuclei of the thalamus.

The several human subjects whose septal areas were stimulated had feelings of pleasure or a "brightening of their attitude." They giggled, talked more, and expressed themselves more freely when the current was on.

Shocks from electrodes within the "punishing centers" evoke behavioral patterns to which monkeys grimace, quiver, and shake. They bite and tear objects with their mouths, their eyes dilate, and their hair stands on end. If stimulated for hours, the monkey becomes irritable, refuses to eat, and may become ill. These effects can be eliminated by stimulating a "pleasure center."

Klüver-Bucy Syndrome

Monkeys with the anterior temporal lobe ablated bilaterally (*Klüver-Bucy syndrome*) exhibit a constellation of emotional expressions. With this loss of the amygdaloid body, uncus, anterior temporal cortex, and parts of hippocampal formation, the animal is apparently released ("release phenomenon") from expressing fear. Wild and aggressive monkeys become tame and docile. The marked absence of emotional responses, such as anger or fear, is accompanied by loss of the facial expressions and vocal protests usually noticed. Formerly fearful monkeys will pick up a live snake or mouse and handle these animals without fear. Hypersexual behavior is marked, with manifestations of autosexual, homosexual, and heterosexual activities.

Memory

The limbic lobe, especially the amygdaloid body and hippocampal formation, has been implicated in the memory for recent events. Human subjects with bilateral lesions of the amygdaloid body–hippocampal region of the temporal lobes retain memory of events prior to the surgical operation (long-term memory). Subsequent to the operation, they may forget any information obtained 10 or so minutes previously. They are unable to commit anything to memory. Lesions are found in the hippocampal formation in some cases of senile dementia. Patients with hippocampal lesions in the dominant hemisphere may have mild disturbances of memory. This may be related to *Korsakoff's syndrome*, in which there is loss of recent memory and sense of time accompanied by a tendency for the patient to fabricate and become easily confused. For example, the subject forgets the question just asked and may reply with irrelevant answers (called *compensatory confabulation*). The hippocampus may be readily induced into convulsant activity. This suggests that the involvement of the hippocampus and other limbic structures can account for many of the bizarre changes in behavior observed in some patients during psychomotor attacks.

Thalamus

The thalami (dorsal thalami) are a pair of egg-shaped masses of gray matter located in the cerebrum central and ventromedial to the cerebral hemispheres (Fig. 20.1). The general conformation of each thalamus roughly follows that of the overlying cerebral cortex. From this central location, the thalamocortical fibers project and radiate three-dimensionally distally through the internal capsule and corona radiata to the cerebral cortex. The thalamus is the hub of the radiation to the cortex.

The thalamus is the final nuclear station where ascending influences are processed before being transmitted to the cerebral cortex. All sensory pathways, except the olfactory pathways, have direct projections to and from thalamic nuclei. The thalamus is the structure where the conscious awareness of crude sensations of pain, touch, and temperature is probably initially realized. It has significant functional roles in the ascending reticular system, in several circuits subserving motor activities (viz., as a link between the cerebellum and cerebral cortex and as a link between the globus pallidus and cerebral cortex), in the limbic system, and in several aspects of the highest expressions of the cerebral cortex.

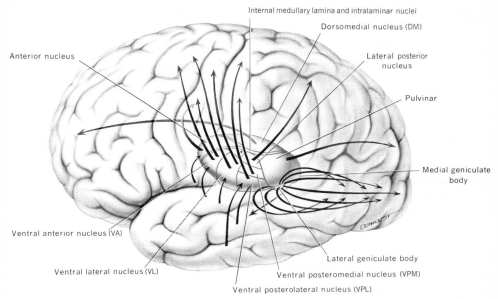

Internal medullary lamina and intralaminar nuclei

Dorsomedial nucleus (DM)

Anterior nucleus

Lateral posterior nucleus

Pulvinar

Medial geniculate body

Ventral anterior nucleus (VA)

Ventral lateral nucleus (VL)

Lateral geniculate body

Ventral posteromedial nucleus (VPM)

Ventral posterolateral nucleus (VPL)

Figure 20.1 Diagram of the thalamus illustrating its major nuclei and some major cortical projections. Many nuclei have reciprocal connections (corticothalamic projections indicated by arrows) with the cortex. The medial geniculate body projects to auditory areas 41 and 42; the lateral geniculate body to visual area 17; the VPM nucleus to the sensory postcentral gyrus (face region of areas 1, 2, and 3) and secondary sensory area; the VPL nucleus to the sensory postcentral gyrus (body region of areas 1, 2, and 3) and secondary sensory area; the VL nucleus to motor areas 4 and 6; the VA nucleus to motor areas 6 and 8 and the orbitofrontal cortex; the anterior nucleus to the limbic cortex; the lateral nucleus and pulvinar (with reciprocal connections) to the association cortex of the parietal and occipitotemporal cortex; and the dorsomedial nucleus (with reciprocal connections) to the prefrontal cortex.

DIVISIONS OF THALAMUS AND INTERNAL CAPSULE

The structural and functional organization of this incompletely understood, complex, integrating station of the nervous system may be obtained by an appreciation of some of the anatomic and physiologic aspects of the following subdivisions (Figs. 20.1 and 20.2). The thalamus is located between the third ventricle medially and the posterior limb of the internal capsule laterally. The *reticular nucleus* is a thin laminar structure on the lateral and ventral surface (abuts against the internal capsule); this nucleus is derived from the ventral thalamus with which it is anatomically continuous. The *nuclei of the midline* (periventricular nuclei), located on the medial surface adjacent to the third ventricle, and the *intralaminar nuclei,* located within the internal medullary lamina, are often grouped together. The diagonally oriented *internal medullary lamina* divides the thalamus into a *lateral group of nuclei* and a *medial* (actually posteromedial) *group of nuclei.* The lateral

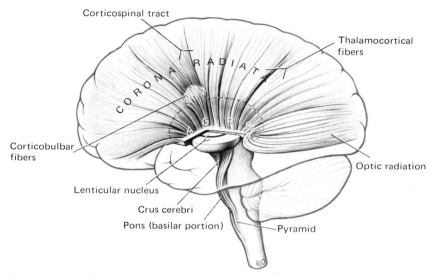

Corticospinal tract

Thalamocortical fibers

Corticobulbar fibers

Optic radiation

Lenticular nucleus

Crus cerebri

Pons (basilar portion)

Pyramid

Figure 20.2 Schematic representation of some component fiber tracts of the internal capsule and their cortical projections. A, anterior limb; G, genu; P, posterior limb; R, retrolenticular portion of the posterior limb.

group is, in turn, divided into a *ventral tier* and a *dorsal tier*. The nuclei of the ventral tier comprise the medial geniculate body (MGB; audition), lateral geniculate body (LGB; vision), ventral posterior nucleus (VP; general modalities and taste), ventral lateral nucleus (VL), and ventral anterior nucleus (VA). The nuclei of the dorsal tier comprise the pulvinar and lateral (lateral dorsal and lateral posterior) nuclei. In the rostral end of the thalamus just caudal to the genu of the internal capsule is the anterior nuclear group.

The *medial geniculate body* is divided into the parvocellular (lateral) portion and the magnocellular (medial) portion, called the posterior thalamic zone or region (Fig. 6.1). The *parvocellular portion* is the relay nucleus of the auditory pathway, whereas the *posterior thalamic zone* is intercalated in a general sensory pathway with a role in the perception of pain and noxious stimuli. This zone receives influences from the ipsilateral and contralateral sides of the body via the spinothalamic tract, ascending reticular pathway, and other ascending pathways. The posterior thalamic zone has direct connections with the secondary somatic sensory area of the cortex (Chap. 22).

The major thalamic nuclei have also been classified as specific cortical relay nuclei, specific association nuclei, and nonspecific nuclei. The *specific relay nuclei* receive input from ascending pathways or major subcortical nuclei, and project to and receive projections from restricted cortical areas related to specific functions. These include the lateral and medial geniculate bodies, the ventral posterior, ventral lateral, and part of the ventral anterior (parvocellular portion) nuclei, and the anterior nuclear group. The ascending pathways project to the LGB (optic tract), MGB (lateral lemniscus), and VP nucleus (medial lemniscus, spinothalamic tract, and trigeminothalamic tract). The VL, VA, and anterior nuclear group receive fibers from the cerebellum, red nucleus, globus pallidus, hypothalamus, and mamillary body. The *association nuclei* receive no direct input from the ascending pathways but have reciprocal connections with the association areas of the cortex (Fig. 20.3). These include the pulvinar and the lateral dorsal, lateral posterior, and dorsomedial nuclei. The nonspecific nuclei include the intralaminar, the ventral anterior (magnocellular portion), thalamic reticular nuclei, and nuclei of the midline.

INTERNAL CAPSULE

The internal capsule is one portion of a continuous massive sheet of fibers projecting to, or projecting from, the cerebral cortex; the sheet extends as the crus cerebri of the midbrain, internal capsule (located between thalamus and nuclei of the corpus striatum), and corona radiata of the white matter and the cerebral cortex (see Chap. 1 and Figs. 1.5, 11.4, 11.5, and 20.2).

The fibers passing through the *anterior* (*caudatolenticular*) *limb* of the internal capsule include: (1) frontopontine fibers to nuclei in pons, (2) corticostriate fibers to striatum, and the following pathways composed of reciprocal connections of fibers interconnecting (3) prefrontal cortex with dorsomedial thalamic nucleus, (4) cingulate gyrus and anterior thalamic nucleus, and (5) septal area and hypothalamus (medial forebrain bundle).

The *genu* of the internal capsule contains corticobulbar and corticoreticular fibers.

The *posterior* (*thalamolenticular*) *limb* is composed of both motor pathways and sensory pathways. Through the rostral half of this limb pass the corticospinal and rubrospinal tracts. Through the caudal half of this limb pass thalamocortical projections from the ventral anterior, ventral lateral, and ventral posterior thalamic nuclei.

The *retrolenticular* (*postlenticular*) *portion* of the posterior limb is composed of optic (geniculocalcarine) radiation, auditory (geniculotemporal) radiation, and corticopontine fibers from the temporal, parietal, and occipital cortices.

NUCLEI OF THE THALAMUS[1] (Fig. 20.1)
Reticular Nucleus

The *reticular nucleus* of the thalamus receives its main input from the cerebral cortex and other thalamic nuclei; it projects its output primarily to

---

[1]The nomenclature of some thalamic nuclei is confusing; for example, the ventral lateral nucleus (VL) is also called the *nucleus ventralis lateralis* or the *lateral ventral nucleus*. The names in this account are adopted because their use is gaining acceptance in the literature.

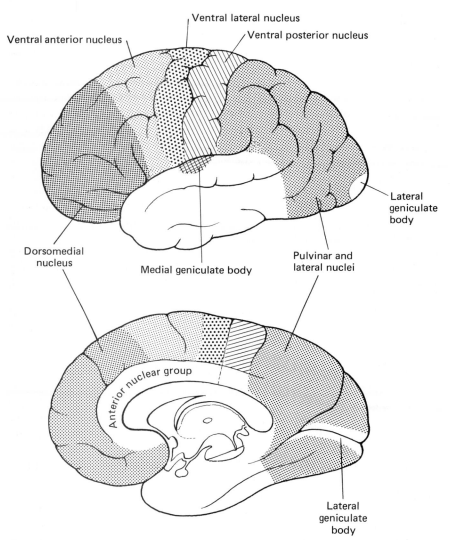

Figure 20.3 Lateral and medial views of the left cerebral hemisphere illustrating cortical projection areas of the thalamic nuclei.

both specific and nonspecific thalamic nuclei and to the midbrain tegmentum. It probably serves to integrate intrathalamic activities; it is not considered to be a part of the reticular system.

Periventricular and Intralaminar Nuclei

The *periventricular nuclei* of the midline and the *intralaminar thalamic nuclei* are integrated into the reticular system. In the caudal aspect of the internal medullary lamina in the middle third of the thalamus are (1) the *centro-median nucleus,* located between the ventral posterior and dorsomedial thalamic nuclei, and (2) the *parafascicular nucleus,* located medial to the centromedian nucleus in the vicinity of the habenulopeduncular fasciculus (tract). These two nuclei and the rostrally located paracentral, central medial, and central lateral nuclei are the nonspecific intralaminar thalamic nuclei, which receive their main input from (1) brainstem reticular formation (ascending reticular system) and (2) other thalamic nuclei. In addition, the centromedian nucleus receives input from the globus pallidus, the rostral nuclei from the cerebellum, and the parafascicular and rostral intralaminar nuclei from the spinothalamic tract and spinoreticulothalamic pathway. The efferent influences from these nuclei project (1) profusely and topograph-ically (point-to-point) upon the neostriatum (caudate nucleus and putamen), (2) sparsely and diffusely (not point-to-point) to the entire neocortex, and (3) to some other thalamic nuclei. Direct connections from these nuclei to the cortex apparently can now be demonstrated. These diffuse projections to the cortex are, in all likelihood, collateral fibers of the axons projecting to the neostriatum. These cortical projections have a significant role in the function of the reticular system (Chap. 14).

The small group of nuclei of the midline are probably concerned with visceral activities; they have connections with the dorsomedial thalamic nucleus and the thalamic intralaminar nuclei.

Ventral Tier of Thalamic Nuclei (Figs. 20.1 and 20.3)

The nuclei of the *ventral tier* comprise (from caudal to rostral) the *lateral geniculate body (LGB), medial geniculate body (MGB), ventral posterior lateral (VPL)* and *ventral posterior medial (VPM) nuclei, ventral lateral (VL) nu-cleus,* and *ventral anterior (VA) nucleus.* The medial and lateral geniculate bodies (nuclei) are called the *metathalamus.*

The *lateral geniculate body* (1) receives input from both eyes via retino-fugal fibers of the optic tract and possibly from the visual cortex via cortico-geniculate fibers, and (2) projects to the visual cortex via the geniculo-calcarine tract (optic radiation). Internuclear connections with the pulvinar are present.

The *medial geniculate body* (parvocellular part) (1) receives influences from both ears via the fibers of the brachium of the inferior colliculus (lateral lemniscus) and from the auditory cortex (transverse gyri of Heschl, areas 41 and 42), and (2) projects to the primary auditory cortex via the auditory radiation, descending fibers to the inferior colliculus, and other fibers to the pulvinar. The *anterior* or *magnocellular part* of the MGB, also called the *posterior thalamic region,* receives input from the spinothalamic tract, medial lemniscus, inferior colliculus, and ascending reticular pathways (polysensory input); this part is related to the adjacent PVL thalamic nucleus. This region projects to the secondary somatic sensory area (Chap. 22).

The *ventral posterior nucleus* (makes up much of the so-called *ventrobasal complex*), the nucleus of termination for the general sensory and gustatory pathways, is subdivided into a ventroposterolateral (VPL) and ventroposteromedial (VPM) nuclei. The VPL nucleus is the nucleus of termination of the lateral spinothalamic tract (pain and thermal sense from the body), medial lemniscus (touch, deep sensibility, and vibratory sense from the body), and anterior spinothalamic tract (light touch from the body). The VPM nucleus is the nucleus of termination of the taste pathways from the nucleus solitarius and of trigeminothalamic tracts (general sensory modalities from the head). A somatotopic distribution is represented as follows: The pathways from the lower extremity terminate in the posterolateral aspect, from body segments in the intermediate location, and from the upper extremity in the anteromedial aspect of the VPL nucleus. The modalities are topographically localized within the VPM nucleus; taste is projected to the medial portion of the nucleus, tactile sense to the lateral portion, and temperature to the intermediate portion. The VP nucleus has precise point-to-point projections to the primary somesthetic cortex (postcentral gyrus, areas 1, 2, and 3). This is consistent with the somatotopic organization of this cortical area and with the modality-specific cortical neurons. In addition, the VP nucleus probably has connections with somatic sensory area II. As in the other ascending systems, descending influences from the postcentral gyrus are projected to the VP nucleus.

The *ventral lateral nucleus* (VL) is an integral nucleus in the feedback circuits of (1) cerebral cortex to cerebellar cortex back to cerebral cortex (Fig. 15.3), and (2) cerebral cortex to basal ganglia to thalamus to cerebral cortex (Fig. 21.1). The VL receives a major input from the dentate nucleus of the contralateral cerebellar hemisphere (dentatothalamic tract) and red nucleus (dentatorubrothalamic tract), and important input from the ipsilateral globus pallidus via the thalamic fasciculus and the substantia nigra. There is apparently an overlap of the input from the dentate nucleus and globus pallidus before powerful influences of the VL upon motor activity are exerted. The VL has somatotopically organized reciprocal connections with the precentral motor cortex (area 4): the medial region of VL with the cortical face area; the intermediate region with the arm and body area; and the lateral region with the leg area. Through the projection to the motor cortex, the VL exerts its role as the main subcortical gateway to and prime mover of the motor pathways. Lesions in the VL may ameliorate the contralateral tremors and rigidity in patients with Parkinson's disease.

The *ventral anterior nucleus* (VA) has a dual role as a specific thalamic nucleus and as a nonspecific thalamic nucleus of the reticular system. The input is derived from the globus pallidus (fibers pass via ansa lenticularis and lenticular fasciculus to the principle part), substantia nigra (fibers terminate in the magnocellular part), brainstem reticular formation, intralaminar nuclei, nuclei of the midline, and collateral branches of descending fibers from the cerebral cortex. The influences relating to somatic motor mechanisms are relayed to the premotor (area 6) cortex (Fig. 21.1). The nonspecific input from the intralaminar thalamic nuclei to nonspecific portion of VA are processed and projected to the orbital cerebral cortex (Chap. 19).

Dorsal Tier of Thalamic Nuclei

The dorsal tier of the lateral nuclear group comprises the lateral dorsal (LD), lateral posterior (LP), and the pulvinar nuclear complex (Figs. 20.1 and 20.3).

The *LD nucleus* is a posterior extension of the anterior nuclear group. Its connections are not well understood. Input is derived from the mamillary bodies via the mamillothalamic tract. Its efferent projections are mainly to the cingulate gyrus of the limbic lobe. Reciprocal connections with the posterior parietal association cortex (precuneus) on the medial aspect of the hemisphere probably exist. The nucleus is primarily integrated into the limbic system (Chap. 19).

The LP and pulvinar nuclei have extensive reciprocal connections with the association neocortex on the medial and lateral aspects of the parietal and occipital lobes. The LP nucleus, located caudal to the LD, probably receives its major input from the primary relay nuclei including the MGB, LGB, and VP nuclei. Reciprocal connections are made with superior parietal cortex (areas 5 and 7). The pulvinar is a large nuclear mass overhanging the geniculate bodies; it is divisible into several nuclei. Their major input is derived from the MGB, LGB, superior colliculus, and VP nuclei. Reciprocal connections are made with the association cortex of the parietal, posterior temporal, and nonstriate occipital lobes. In a general way the dorsal tier nuclei (LD, LP, and pulvinar) have reciprocal connections with association cortex of the occipital, parietal, and posterior temporal lobes on both lateral and medial surfaces (no connections are made with primary sensory areas—primary sensory areas 1, 2, and 3, primary auditory area 41, and primary visual area 17).

Anterior Nuclear Group of the Thalamus (Fig. 20.1)

The anterior group of nuclei, comprising the anteroventral, anterodorsal, and anteromedial nuclei, forms the *anterior thalamic tubercle*. They are integrated into the circuitry of the limbic system (Chap. 19). The anterior nuclei have (1) reciprocal connections with the hypothalamus, particularly the mamillary body, via the fibers of the mamillothalamic tract, and (2) some input via the fornix. In turn, nuclei of these areas have reciprocal connections with the mesocortex of the cingulate gyrus.

Dorsomedial (Medial) Nucleus

The massive *dorsomedial (DM, medial) nucleus,* located between the internal medullary lamina and the third ventricle, is divided into a *magnocellular* (*large cell*) *portion* and a larger *parvocellular* (*small cell*) *portion.* The nucleus has rich connections with the intralaminar nuclei, including the nuclei of the midline and the centromedian nucleus, and the various thalamic nuclei of the lateral group. The magnocellular portion has connections (many are reciprocal) with the amygdaloid body, lateral hypothalamus, and the temporal and caudal orbitofrontal neocortex. The parvocellular portion has massive topically organized reciprocal connections with the prefrontal cortex (areas 9, 10, 11, and 12—all rostral to area 6). The DM nucleus probably acts to integrate certain influences from somatic and visceral sources and, in conjunction with the prefrontal cortex, has roles in the various expressions of feeling tone, affect, emotion, and behavior. Some changes in these expressions are often noted in patients following psychosurgery (prefrontal lobotomy, leukotomy).

FUNCTIONAL CONSIDERATIONS

The thalamus is a major neural processor and integrator involved in essentially all activities of the forebrain. All general and special sensory systems, except the olfactory system, project their major input to the thalamus before the processed information is relayed to the cerebral cortex. The nuclei of the midline, intralaminar nuclei, and part of the ventral anterior nucleus are essential in the reticular system as linkages in the circuitry between the brainstem reticular pathways and the other thalamic nuclei, higher centers of the limbic lobe (and system), and the neocortex. Thalamic output is the chief source of input to the cerebral cortex and to the basal ganglia; these connections are, to a large degree, integrated into intracerebral circuits including (1) reciprocal connections between thalamic nuclei and the cerebral cortex and (2) the cortex–basal ganglia–thalamus–cortex circuit (Chap. 21). In addition, intrathalamic integration occurs through the interconnections and interactions between the nonspecific nuclei and the specific thalamic nuclei. The thalamus has a basic role in somatic motor activity through its strategically located nuclei (VA and VL), which receive input from the cerebellum and basal ganglia (directly from globus pallidus) and project influences to the motor cortex.

The thalamus has a significant role in the conscious appreciation of sensation. The general aspects of crude sensory modalities (pain, touch, temperature discrimination, and possibly sound detection) are brought to conscious level in the thalamus. The finer sensory discriminations (those of the somesthetic, visual, auditory, and gustatory senses), which are elevated to the conscious sphere in the cerebral cortex, require the input of the information processed in thalamic nuclei for their final resolution. The conscious appreciation of discriminatory sensations takes place at both thalamic and cortical levels.

The "affective" domain of sensory appreciation is apparently mediated through the thalamic reticular system, dorsomedial nucleus, and anterior nuclear group. The *affect* of an individual relates to his emotional tone and somewhat to the phase of the sleep-wake cycle. Well-being, malaise, and a state of contentment are expressions of affect. The degree of agreeableness or disagreeableness of any stimulus depends on the state of an individual. The same objective degree of pain, temperature, or touch can evoke a remarkable variety of subjective degrees of reactivities. This variety is an expression of affective sensory mechanisms.

Through the functional interaction of the nonspecific nuclei and specific nuclei, the thalamus exerts a regulatory drive upon the cerebral cortex. The thalamic reticular system acts as a modulator and modifier of thalamic processing. In addition, the synchronization and desynchronization of thalamic activity are considered to be dependent, in part, upon recurrent collateral branches of thalamic neurons feeding back on interneurons; in turn, these connections modulate the neurons projecting to the cortex. The thalamus is essential to such expressions of synchrony (or desynchrony) as (1) the rhythmic brain wave activity observed in an EEG and (2) the phasic and tonic movements mediated by the motor pathways. The thalamus is considered to be a "prime mover" of motor pathways. The modulatory effects are exerted in concert with the VL and VA nuclei through (1) the cerebello-thalamocortical pathway (Chap. 21), and (2) the globus pallido–thalamo-cortical pathway (Chap. 21). Through integrative, modulatory, and synchronizing activities, the thalamus exerts a major effect upon the motor expressions via the cerebral cortex and its projection pathways, including the corticospinal, corticorubrospinal, corticostriate, and corticoreticulospinal tracts, among others.

THALAMIC LESIONS

Lesions of the thalamus (as a consequence of vascular impairment) may produce signs known as the *thalamic syndrome*. All general somatic modalities may be diminished on the contralateral half of the head and body without complete anesthesia (lesion of VP nucleus), all general modalities from the face may be normal (VPM not damaged), tactile sense from the face may be intact (bilateral projections from principal trigeminal nucleus), and some pain and temperature sense on the contralateral side may be retained (these modalities may be bilaterally represented in the thalamus or some qualities of these modalities may be felt in the midbrain). In this syndrome, the threshold for pain, temperature, and tactile sensations is usually raised on the side contralateral to the lesion. In addition to the diminution of sensations, mild stimuli may evoke disagreeable sensations (dysesthesias). The feelings elicited from a pinprick may be an intolerable burning and agonizing pain. Heat, cold, and pressure from one's clothes can be exceedingly uncomfortable. Intractable pain, which does not respond to analgesics, may be a consequence. Affect qualities such as compression and numbness are exaggerated during emotional stress. The application of a warm object to the hand may be pleasurable.

These highly overactive sensory responses are probably the result of alterations in frequencies and patterns of input to the thalamus, irritation of injured neurons, and changes in the quality of the output to the cerebral cortex. In addition, the release from some cortical influences upon the thalamus may be contributory (release phenomena).

A neocerebellar lesion results in cerebellar dyskinesia. This is an expression of a release phenomenon, in which the VL nucleus is released from the normal cerebellar influences relayed rhythmically through the dentato-thalamic pathway. Without these influences, the abnormal movements are expressed. The amelioration of cerebellar dyskinesias in man may occur following a surgically placed lesion in the contralateral VL nucleus.

Chapter 21

Basal Ganglia and Extrapyramidal System

The brain exerts a significant role in somatic motor activities through several descending pathways which have been arbitrarily divided into the pyramidal system and the extrapyramidal system. This implies that all descending tracts, their nuclei, and feedback circuits influencing somatic motor movements and responses with the exception of the pyramidal system are included in the extrapyramidal system. Many authorities contend that the term *extrapyramidal system* should be abandoned because of (1) the difficulty in delineating and defining the system precisely (except by exclusion from the pyramidal system), and (2) the fact that the two systems interact and supplement each other. The corticospinal tract is a direct link from the cerebral cortex to the spinal cord. In contrast, the extrapyramidal system conveys its influences from the cerebral cortex and other nuclear complexes to the spinal cord via multineuronal and multisynaptic linkages. Some of the extrapyramidal circuits from the cerebral cortex are integrated into circuits with feedback loops to the cerebral cortex.

The extrapyramidal system includes, among other components, the cerebral cortex; the telencephalic basal ganglia (mainly putamen, caudate

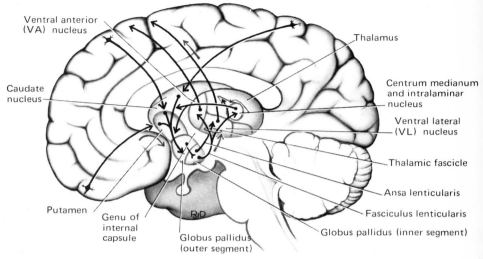

Figure 21.1 Diagram illustrating some of the major interconnections of the "extrapy-ramidal system" involving the cerebral cortex, basal ganglia, thalamus, and brainstem. Arrows indicate major direction of projections.

nucleus, and globus pallidus); other subcortical nuclei of the diencephalon (subthalamic nucleus), midbrain (red nucleus and substantia nigra), and pons and medulla (nuclei in the reticular formation); some closed or feed-back circuits (noted below); and a number of tracts and pathways including the corticorubrospinal and corticoreticulospinal pathways (Fig. 21.1). The cerebellum and its pathways are generally not included (Fig. 15.3).

The extrapyramidal system has a long phylogenetic history; many of its basic elements are present in nonmammalian vertebrates. The pyramidal system is well-developed in mammals. In general, the extrapyramidal system regulates stereotyped movements of a reflex nature, whereas the pyramidal system is involved with the initiation of movements, particularly the skilled, volitional movements of the fingers and of the face. The pyramidal system includes corticobulbar fibers and corticospinal fibers influencing the brain-stem and spinal cord motor nuclei. In this discussion, the basal ganglia include: (1) globus pallidus (pallidum, paleostriatum), (2) striatum (corpus striatum, neostriatum, which includes the caudate nucleus and putamen), and (3) amygdaloid complex [amygdaloid body, archistriatum (Chap. 19)]. The putamen and the globus pallidus form the lenticular nucleus.

CONNECTIONS AND CIRCUITS

The cerebral cortex, basal ganglia, and related nuclei are organized into complex linkages of interconnections, feedback circuits, and descending pathways. The following schemata outline some of the major proposed circuits of the extrapyramidal motor system (Figs. 21.1 through 21.6).

Circuit 1

Cerebral cortex → striatum → globus pallidus → thalamus → cerebral cortex (Figs. 21.1, 21.5, and 21.6).

Widespread areas of the cerebral cortex project corticostriate fibers in a topographically organized arrangement to the ipsilateral striatum (both caudate nucleus and putamen). In turn, fibers from the striatum terminate topographically in the globus pallidus. From the medial pallidal segment fibers course via the *ansa lenticularis* (loops under the internal capsule) and *fasciculus lenticularis* (penetrates through internal capsule); these fascicles join to form the *thalamic fasciculus* before terminating in the VA, VL, and centrum medianum (CM) nuclei of the thalamus. The VA and VL nuclei project somatotopically to the premotor cortex (areas 6 and 8) and to the motor cortex (area 4).

Other connections of the nuclear centers of this circuit add to the complexity. The CM nucleus (which receives input from the globus pallidus) and other intralaminar thalamic nuclei project to the striatum: the CM projects to the putamen, and other intralaminar nuclei project to the caudate nucleus. In a sense the CM nucleus is incorporated in a closed circuit relaying

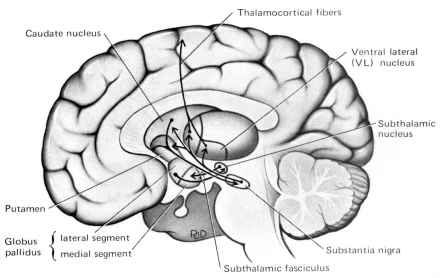

Figure 21.2 Diagram illustrating some of the major circuits of the "extrapyramidal system." The nigrostriatal (substantia nigra to striatum) fibers compose the dopamine neuronal pathway. Arrows indicate major direction of projections.

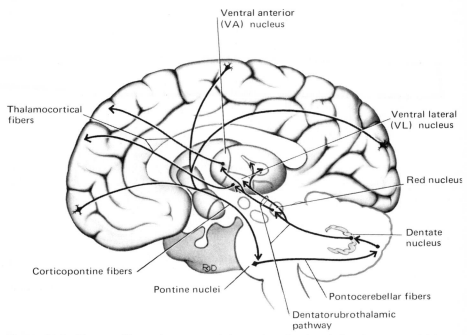

Figure 21.3 Diagram illustrating some of the major circuits of the "extrapyramidal system." Arrows indicate major direction of projections.

back to the striatum. In addition, the globus pallidus projects pallidotegmental fibers to the pedunculopontine tegmental nucleus (lower midbrain) and possibly other brainstem reticular nuclei.

Circuit 2

This circuit (Figs. 21.2, 21.4, and 21.6) involves the substantia nigra. It comprises the following sequences: (1) Cerebral cortex to the striatum to the substantia nigra. The striatonigral fibers project to both the pars compacta and pars reticularis of the substantia nigra. (2) The projections from the substantia nigra, directed rostrally via (a) nigrostriatal fibers to the striatum, or (b) nigrothalamic fibers to the VA and VL thalamic nuclei, which project to the motor and premotor cortical areas. Direct corticonigral fibers probably do not exist.

The substantia nigra is divided into the anteriorly located pars reticularis (adjacent to the crus cerebri) and the posteriorly located pars compacta. The *pars reticularis* is rich in iron and lacking in melanin pigment. The *pars compacta* contains neurons rich in dopamine (a catecholamine) and melanin.

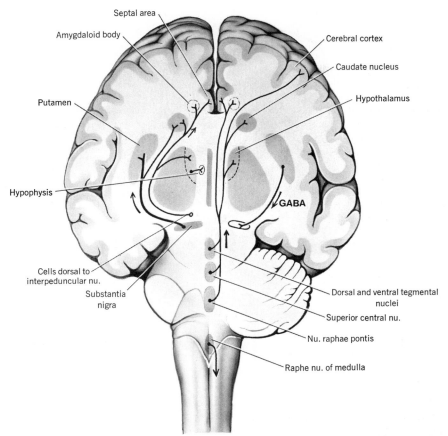

Septal area

Amygdaloid body

Cerebral cortex

Caudate nucleus

Putamen

Hypothalamus

Hypophysis

GABA

Cells dorsal to
interpeduncular nu.

Substantia
nigra

Dorsal and ventral tegmental
nuclei

Superior central nu.

Nu. raphae pontis

Raphe nu. of medulla

Figure 21.4 The dopaminergic pathways (left) and the serotoninergic (5-HT) pathway (right). GABA neurons are indicated on the right. These pathways are described in the text. nu, nuclei.

Reciprocal topographic projections apparently are the main interconnections (1) between the pars reticularis and the VA and VL thalamic nuclei and (2) between the pars compacta and the striatum. The substantia nigra does not project caudally. The nigral efferent projections to the VA and VL thalamic nuclei terminate in different regions of these thalamic nuclei than those projections from the globus pallidus (no overlap). The nigrostriatal fibers compose the *dopamine neuronal system;* the substantia nigra, nigrostriatal fibers, and striatum are rich in dopamine, which may be an active neurotransmitter. The striatonigral fibers contain the putative neurotransmitter gamma butyric acid (GABA). See "Functional Considerations" below.

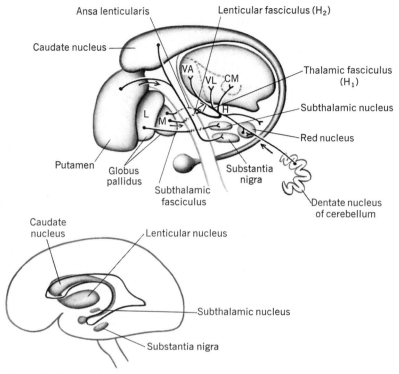

Figure 21.5 Lower: The location of the basal ganglia with reference to the lateral ventricle. Upper: The fields of Forel (H, H_1 and H_2) and some efferent projections of basal ganglia and cerebellum. The pallidofugal fibers pass through three bundles: ansa lenticularis, lenticular fasciculus (H_2), and subthalamic fasciculus. The former two bundles and the cerebellar projections join in the H field of Forel (prerubral field) and continue as the thalamic fasciculus (H_1) to various thalamic nuclei. CM, centromedian nucleus; H, the H field of Forel; L and M, lateral and medial segments of the globus pallidus; VA, ventral anterior thalamic nucleus; VL, ventral lateral thalamic nucleus; ZI, zona incerta.

Circuit 3

The *subthalamic nucleus* is integrated in the above circuitry (Fig. 21.2). Fibers from the lateral segment of the globus pallidus terminate in the subthalamus, which, in turn, projects back to the medial segment of the globus pallidus. These fibers form the subthalamic fasciculus, which passes through the internal capsule (Figs. 21.5, 21.6).

Circuit 4

Another circuit influences the extrapyramidal system. Its sequence includes the cerebral cortex → ipsilateral pontine nuclei (corticopontine fibers) →

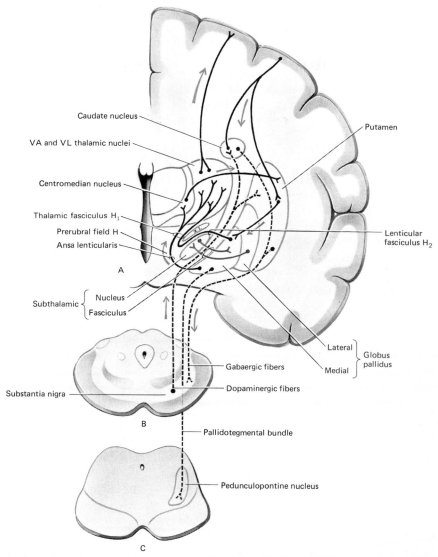

Caudate nucleus

VA and VL thalamic nuclei

Centromedian nucleus

Thalamic fasciculus H₁

Prerubral field H

Ansa lenticularis

A

Subthalamic { Nucleus / Fasciculus

Substantia nigra

B

Putamen

Lenticular fasciculus H₂

Lateral ⎫
         ⎬ Globus
Medial ⎭ pallidus

Gabaergic fibers

Dopaminergic fibers

Pallidotegmental bundle

Peduncolopontine nucleus

C

Figure 21.6 Diagram of the major circuits of the "extrapyramidal system" illustrated (A) in a coronal section through the cerebrum and (B and C) transverse sections through the upper and lower midbrain. Of the pallidofugal projections, the ansa lenticularis is most rostral, the lenticular fasciculus is intermediate, and the subthalamic fasciculus is the most caudal in location. Note the pallidofugal fibers (pallidotegmental bundle) to the peduncolopontine nucleus. The nigrostriatal fibers are dopaminergic while the striatonigral fibers are gabanergic (GABA). ZI, zona incerta.

contralateral cerebellar cortex (pontocerebellar fibers) → dentate nucleus of cerebellum → contralateral VL, VA, and intralaminar thalamic nuclei (dentatothalamic fibers) → cerebral cortex (areas 4, 6, and 8) (Figs. 15.4 and 21.3).

There is an overlapping of the dentatothalamic fibers from the cerebellum and pallidothalamic fibers from the globus pallidus in the VL thalamic nucleus. Some influences from the cerebellum to the thalamus are also conveyed via the dentatorubrothalamic pathway (see Chap. 15, "Cerebellum").

Circuit 5

The extrapyramidal subcortical influences upon the cerebral cortex are, in turn, projected from the cerebral cortex to the brainstem and spinal cord motor nuclei via several descending pathways (Figs. 9.1 and 9.2). These include the pyramidal pathways (corticospinal and corticobulbar tracts), corticorubrospinal pathways, corticoreticular pathway, and corticoreticulospinal pathway (medial and lateral reticulospinal tracts).

FUNCTIONAL CONSIDERATIONS

The extrapyramidal system is functionally organized into an exquisitely tuned complex of interconnected nuclei. The role of the basal ganglia and associated nuclei is to modulate motor activities through circuits which directly and indirectly feed back to the cerebral cortex. In turn, the cortex projects its influences to the brainstem and spinal levels through the descending pathways upon the alpha and gamma motor neurons. The malfunction of various nuclear complexes results in an imbalance in the interactions within the complex circuitry of the extrapyramidal system. This is a plausible explanation for the variety and assortment of symptoms and signs noted in the clinically observed disorders in the control of posture and movements when the harmonious interactions are altered within this system. Posture is modified by an increase in muscle tone to a similar degree in the agonists and antagonists of a muscle group without an accompanying increase in reflex activity; this is called *rigidity*. The abnormal involuntary movements, called *dyskinesias*, may be rhythmic or arrhythmic, generally without paralysis of the muscles. The motor disorders resulting from the improper functioning of the extrapyramidal system, the basal ganglia, and associated nuclei include paralysis agitans (Parkinson's disease), athetosis, choreas, and ballism.

Paralysis agitans (*Parkinson's disease*) is characterized by rigidity and tremor. The rigidity is essentially the same in all muscles; it is accompanied by poverty of movements but normal deep tendon reflex activity. As a limb is passively forced through flexor or extensor movements, the muscular resistance alternately increases and decreases to give a cogwheel effect. From a standing position, the patient has difficulty in taking his initial steps. The subject also has the same problem in arresting the movement. During forward locomotion, short, shuffling steps are taken. The "masked" face has a fixed expression accompanied by no overt spontaneous emotional response. The tremor, with its regular frequency and amplitude, occurs while the subject is at rest; it is lost or reduced during a movement. Degenerative changes in the globus pallidus and substantia nigra are present in Parkinsonian patients; in addition there is a marked reduction to absence of dopamine in the substantia nigra and striatum. Surgical lesions in the globus pallidus or ventral lateral thalamic nucleus may reduce or abolish the tremor and rigidity. L-*dopa* (L-dihydroxyphenylalanine) in low doses may ameliorate the rigidity and in high doses may decrease the tremor. L-dopa is a common precursor of melanin and dopamine. This rigidity is associated with the increased tonic stretch reflexes; it may be due to the increased activity of the static gamma fusiform system (Chap. 5).

The movements of *athetosis* are slow and are exaggerated by voluntary movement. The slow, writhing character of the involuntary movement of the extremities appears wormlike. The alternating adduction and abduction of the shoulder joint is accompanied by flexion and extension of the wrist and fingers. Usually the wrist is flexed, and the fingers hyperextended. Grimaces of the face may occur during the limb movements. This dyskinesia may be due to a lesion in the striatum, mainly in the putamen, following the trauma of a birth injury. Such injury suggests that the striatum has an inhibitory role.

Choreas (dances) are characterized by jerky, irregular, brisk, graceful movements of the limbs accompanied by involuntary twitchings of the face. These movements are expressed primarily by the distal segments of the extremities. In advanced cases, the patient is almost always in motion when awake. There is no reduction in muscle power. *Huntington's chorea* is a hereditary form, which becomes progressively worse with age after its initial appearance, often in the late thirties. Damage to the striatum and the cerebral cortex are presumed to be casual.

The neuronal loop (Figs. 21.4 and 21.6) of (1) dopaminergic (DA) neurons of the substantia nigra projecting to the neostriatum (Chap. 11, "Dopaminergic Pathway"), (2) cholinergic interneurons of neostriatum, and (3) neostriatal neurons projecting back to the substantia nigra (strionigral fibers) has been implicated in some dyskinesias. The nigrostriatal DA system releases DA in the neostriatum to inhibit the activity of the cholinergic interneurons. These interneurons release acetylcholine which exerts excitatory influences on the strionigral neurons, which exert inhibitory influences on the DA neurons in the substantia nigra. The strionigral neurons release gamma-aminobutyric acid (GABA), which is the putative inhibitory neurotransmitter. In paralysis agitans (Parkinson's disease) there is marked reduction to depletion of DA in the substantia nigra and neostriatum (Fig.

21.6). Patients with Huntington's chorea exhibit a measurable decrease in GABA in the strionigral neurons (Fig. 21.6).

Ballism ("throwing") is characterized by violent, abnormal, flaillike movements originating mainly from the activity of the proximal appendicular muscles of the shoulder and pelvis. The movements cease during sleep. There is a reduction of muscle tone. These symptoms are exhibited unilaterally with a lesion in the contralateral subthalamic nucleus.

Symptoms associated with the malfunctioning of the basal ganglia are usually observed bilaterally. However, those symptoms on one side result from lesions in the contralateral basal ganglia; this is a consequence of the circuits by which the basal ganglia project to the ipsilateral cerebral cortex, which, in turn, relays its influences via the corticofugal pathways to the contralateral side (i.e., see *ballism* above). The abnormal movements resulting from lesions in the basal ganglia circuitry are an expression of release phenomena, in which the inhibitory influences on such structures as the globus pallidus or ventral lateral nucleus of the thalamus are lost or reduced. Surgical lesions of these "released structures" (globus pallidus and VL) are known to ameliorate the symptoms in many patients. In this context, the loss of dopamine, noted in patients with Parkinsonism, is presumed to account for the reduction or loss of inhibitory influences upon the striatum.

Chapter 22

Cerebral Cortex

The *cerebral cortex* (*pallium*) is the 600-g gray mantle of the cerebrum, composing about 40 percent of the brain by weight. Estimates indicate that the 15 billion cortical neurons weigh about 180 g and the glial cells and blood vessels weigh about 420 g. The cerebral cortex has an essential functional role in consciousness, mental ability, memory, and intellect.

The cortex is subdivided into the phylogenetically older *allocortex* (heterogenetic cortex), composing about 10 percent of the entire cortex, and the phylogenetically more recent *isocortex* (homogenetic cortex). The allocortex includes (1) the *archicortex* (*archipallium*), composed of the hippocampus and dentate gyrus, and (2) the *paleocortex* (*paleopallium*), comprising the olfactory cortex of the piriform lobe and portions of the parahippocampal gyrus. The *isocortex,* also called the *neocortex* (*neopallium*), is the bulk of the cerebral cortex. The cingulate gyrus and portions of the parahippocampal gyrus are often called the *mesocortex* (*juxtallocortex*) because they are intermediate in structure between the allocortex and isocortex. The mesocortex, archicortex, and paleocortex have been called the *limbic lobe* (Fig. 1.3 and Chap. 19). The neocortex has been parceled in

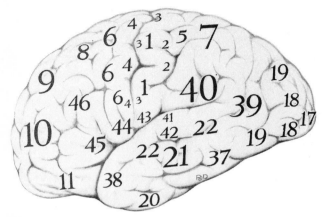

Figure 22.1 Cytoarchitectural map of the lateral surface of the human cerebral cortex, with numbers representing the areas of Brodmann.

several ways; the most commonly used system is the 47 cytoarchitectonic areas of Brodmann (Figs. 22.1 and 22.2), based upon the arrangement of neurons as visualized in Nissl-stained preparations.

ORGANIZATION OF NEOCORTEX

The neocortex is conventionally described as being structurally organized into six horizontal laminae oriented parallel to the cortical surface. However, one of the basic functional units of the cerebral cortex is a physiologically defined vertical column extending from the pial surface to the white matter

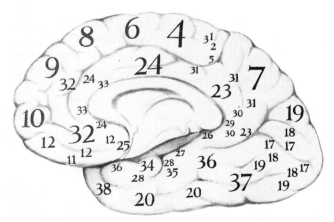

Figure 22.2 Cytoarchitectural map of the medial surface of the human cerebral cortex, with numbers representing the areas of Brodmann.

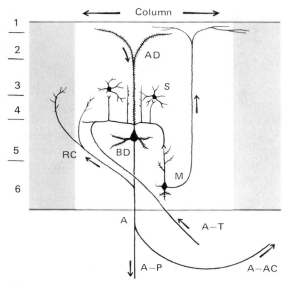

Figure 22.3 Schema of the vertical columnar organization of the cerebral cortex. The basic types of cortical neurons are indicated. A, axon of a pyramidal neuron; A-AC, axon of association or commissural fiber; AD, apical dendrite of a pyramidal neuron; A-P, axon of projection fiber; A-T, axon of neuron in a specific thalamic nucleus; BD, basilar dendrites of a pyramidal neuron; M, Martinotti cell; RC, recurrent collateral branch; S, stellate cell (granule, Golgi type-II cell). Each pyramidal neuron may be an association neuron, commissural neuron, or projection neuron, but not all three. Numbers indicate the six horizontal laminae of the neocortex.

(Fig. 22.3). This *columnar organization* is present in the primary visual cortex (area 17) and primary somesthetic cortex (areas 3, 1, and 2); as yet it has not been demonstrated in all cortical areas. Each of these cortical columns may be (1) a terminus for afferent fibers (input) from other cortical areas and the thalamus, and (2) the source of efferent fibers (output) terminating in other cortical areas of the same hemisphere (association fibers), in the same cortical area of the contralateral hemisphere (commissural fibers passing through the corpus callosum and anterior commissure), and in the subcortical nuclei of the cerebrum, brainstem, and spinal cord (projection fibers). In general, the main receptive layers (input) are laminae I through IV, with lamina IV being the main receptive layer from the specific thalamic nuclei. The main efferent layers (output) are laminae V and VI.

The input to the entire cortex is derived primarily from the thalamus (Chap. 20) and, in part, from the hypothalamus (Chap. 18) and olfactory system (Chap. 19). The output from the neocortex out of the cerebral hemispheres is relayed via the following projection fibers: the corticobulbar and corticoreticular fibers (Chap. 9), corticopontine fibers (Chap. 15), corti-

cothalamic, corticostriate, and corticorubral fibers (Chaps. 20 and 21), and
corticospinal fibers (Chap. 9).

NEURONS OF THE NEOCORTEX

Four basic neuronal cell types are representative of the numerous cortical
neurons (Fig. 22.3). The shape of the cell body and course taken by the axon
are among the criteria used to characterize each cell. Each *pyramidal cell* has
a pyramid-shaped cell body, a branched *apical dendrite* extending toward the
cortical surface, several horizontally directed, branched *basilar dendrites,* and
an *axon* with collateral branches projecting back to the cortex and a main
branch projecting through subcortical white matter. The main axonal
branches of the pyramidal cells comprise the association fibers, commissural
fibers, and projection fibers (listed above). Each *stellate cell* (*granule cell,
Golgi type II cell*) is a multipolar interneuron with a star-shaped body with
short, branched dendrites and a short axon that arborizes and synapses with
other cortical neurons in the immediate vicinity. Each *cell of Martinotti* is a
multipolar interneuron with short, branched dendrites and a branching axon
extending toward the cortical surface and synapsing with other cortical
neurons. The *horizontal cell of Cajal* is a small interneuron of the most
superficial cortical lamina (not present after the circumnatal period); its axon
is oriented parallel to the cortical surface. Except for the pyramidal cells, all
cortical cells are intracortical interneurons.

The input of these columnar units of the neocortex is derived primarily
from other cortical areas and the thalamus. In general, fibers from the
primary thalamic relay nuclei terminate in a rich arborization within laminae
III and IV, while the efferent fibers from other regions terminate in each of
the cortical laminae. The intracortical neuronal circuits are apparently
structured to sustain the vertical columnar organization; the axon collaterals
of the pyramidal cells and the axons of many cortical interneurons are
oriented vertically, while the lateral spread of the axons and dendrites within
the cortex is minimal. Within the complex synaptic connectivity among these
neurons are numerous neuronal chains of small and long loops. The large
numbers of small stellate neurons in man are integrated into a vast number
of loops with an astronomic number of synaptic connections; these neurons
are considered to be "the anatomic expression" of the delicacy of function in
the human brain (Cajal). The output of this intracortical processing is
projected via the axons of the pyramidal neurons. Some axonal fibers are
incorporated into complex intrahemispheric and interhemispheric loops
which integrate the functional activity among different cortical areas of the
same and opposite hemispheres. In addition, complex feedback circuits with
subcortical centers are also integrated in the functional activity of the cortex,
e.g., cerebral cortex → cerebellum → thalamus → cerebral cortex circuit (Fig.

15.3); cerebral cortex → basal ganglia → thalamus → cerebral cortex circuit (Fig. 21.1); and reciprocal connections with thalamic nuclei (Chap. 20).

FUNCTIONAL ASPECTS

The cerebral cortex has been parceled into a number of areas described in terms of several structural and functional criteria. At present, the precise role of the cortex in memory, consciousness, and learning is not understood. The functional aspect of the cortex is interpreted in terms of evidence obtained from the subjectively appreciated experiences and objectively observed physical responses noted in conscious and unconscious subjects (1) who have areas of cortex damaged by lesions or surgical ablation, (2) in whom cortical sites were stimulated electrically, and (3) who have irritative lesions resulting in epileptic seizures.

The cerebral cortex may be subdivided into (1) "sensory areas" includ-

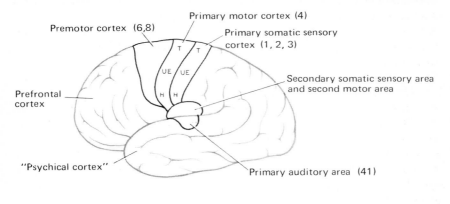

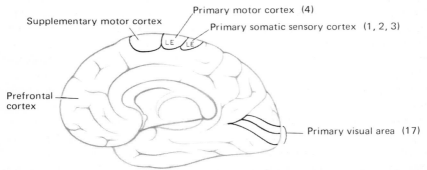

Figure 22.4 The location of several functional areas of the cerebral cortex. The representation of body parts on the primary motor and somatic sensory cortices include the head (H), upper extremity (UE), trunk (T), and lower extremity (LE). Numbers represent areas of Brodmann.

ing primary sensory areas, secondary sensory areas, parasensory association areas, and an "association" area of sensory association areas, (2) "motor areas" including primary motor area, premotor area, and supplementary motor area, and (3) "psychical" and prefrontal association areas (Fig. 22.4).

"SENSORY AREAS"

General Somesthetic Senses

The primary receptive somesthetic cortex (primary sensory area, postcentral gyrus, and its medial extension in the paracentral gyrus, areas 1, 2, and 3 of the parietal lobe, Figs. 20.3 and 22.4) receives input from the ventral posterior nucleus of the thalamus (influences from the opposite side of the body generally). The projection to this area is topographically organized as an upside down sensory homunculus with the head represented ventrally near the lateral sulcus and the lower extremity in the paracentral gyrus. The modality-specific columns in area 1 receive projections concerned with cutaneous and deep sensibility senses, those in area 2 receive projections concerned with deep sensibility, and those in area 3 receive projections concerned with cutaneous senses, e.g., touch and position, pressure, and vibratory senses. Pain and temperature apparently have slight representation in this sensory area.

The secondary somatic area (somatic area II) is located on the superior tip of the lateral fissure ventral to the primary sensory and motor areas (Figs. 20.3 and 22.4). This area is topographically organized with respect to general sensory input including pain from both sides of the body; it is coextensive with second motor area. It receives input from the *posterior thalamic zone*, which, in turn, receives a bilateral input from ascending pathways (Chap. 20). The homunculus of somatic area II is oriented with the head overlapping that of the primary sensory area. Taste is represented in area 43 located in the precentral gyrus adjacent to the lateral sulcus.

Further neural processing of the multisensory somesthetic input takes place before being integrated into the levels where perception of shape, size, and texture and the identification of objects by contact occur (e.g., recognition of an object, such as a key or fork, after handling it). This occurs after information is conveyed for further processing in the association areas of the superior parietal lobule (parasensory areas 5 and 7) and in the supramarginal gyrus (area 40). These areas have well-developed reciprocal connections with the pulvinar of the thalamus. Lesions in area 40 may result in tactile agnosia and tactile aphasia (see below). Functional activity of this area is apparently essential for perception of the general senses.

Visual Sense

The primary visual area (visual area I, striate area 17 in the occipital lobe) is located on both banks of the calcarine sulcus; it is the cortical terminus for the optic radiation from the lateral geniculate body of the thalamus (Chap. 16). The parasensory association visual cortex includes visual area II (area 18) and visual area III (area 19), while the higher association visual cortex is presumed to be the angular gyrus (area 39). Each area represents a higher level of neural processing. Visual area II is a mirror-image representation of visual area I, and visual area III is another representation (Fig. 22.4). Within visual areas II and III are found complex visual cells and hypercomplex visual cells (Chap. 16). The complex cells receive their input from a variety of simple cells of visual area I, while hypercomplex cells probably receive their stimuli from complex cells. Complex cells respond optimally to linear environmental stimuli, while hypercomplex cells respond optimally to curvatures or angular changes in the direction of a line. Lesions in area 39 of the dominant hemisphere may result in the patient's inability to comprehend the symbols of language and express himself through them. Presumably this area is essential to the comprehension of a visual image. These association areas are integrated with the "Psychical Cortex" (see below) and the thalamus (pulvinar) through reciprocal connections. As yet, the manner in which visual images are perceived is unknown.

Auditory Sense

The primary auditory area (transverse gyri of Heschl, area 41, auditory area I of the temporal lobe) is the cortical terminus of the auditory radiations from the medial geniculate body of the thalamus (Chap. 13). This area responds to broad bands of the audible spectrum; it is tonotopically organized. This primary cortex appears to be essential for the detection of changes in frequency and in the orientation of the source of a sound. Auditory area II (area 42) has a higher threshold to sound intensity than the primary cortex. Area 22 of the superior temporal gyrus is the higher association cortex. Patients with lesions of area 22 on the dominant side have profound difficulty in the interpretation of sounds; the spoken language may be meaningless or extremely difficult for them to comprehend.

The cortex of the rostral superior temporal gyrus may subserve a conscious phase of vestibular activity. The feeling of dizziness and rotation, which occurs during direct stimulation of this area, is the justification for calling it the primary vestibular area. It receives projections from the medial geniculate body.

"Association Area" of the Sensory Association Areas

Area 40 (supramarginal gyrus), area 39 (angular gyrus), and area 22 (superior temporal gyrus) are contiguous areas interconnected by association fibers; they appear to be an "association area" of the association sensory areas in that they process neural input from each of the association sensory areas. From this "association area" neural information is relayed via association fibers to motor areas of the frontal lobe where neural programming occurs that is instrumental in the exquisite control of speech, writing, and other highly skilled movements. Influences from these motor areas (areas 4, 6, and 8) are ultimately projected from the cortex via corticobulbar, corticospinal, and other tracts. The functional role of these areas has been inferred mainly from symptoms and signs in patients with lesions in these cortical regions, especially of the dominant hemisphere; the ascending sensory pathways and descending motor pathways are undamaged and are functioning normally in these subjects.

Lesions in these "association areas" show mixtures of symptoms, which have been variously named and defined. In a simple classification the clinical signs may be expressed in the continuous chain of agnosias, aphasias, and apraxias. *Agnosia* is the inability to recognize or to be aware of an object. A *tactile agnosia* (*astereognosis*), inability to recognize familiar objects through senses of touch and proprioception, may result from large lesions in the supramarginal gyrus (area 40) of the dominant hemisphere. A *visual agnosia* (*alexia*), inability to recognize objects by sight, may result from a lesion of the angular gyrus (area 39) of the dominant hemisphere. An *auditory agnosia*, inability to recognize familiar sounds and words, may result from a lesion of area 22 of the dominant hemisphere. *Receptive* (*sensory*) *aphasia* is a defect in ability to symbolize—i.e., inadequacy in the appreciation of the written and spoken word—even though the object is recognized. These aphasias seem to be associated with lesions of the posterior temporoparietal region (areas 22 and 39) of the dominant hemisphere. The patient with a lesion primarily in area 39 may be unable to comprehend the written language; even words written by the patient himself are not recognized as words. The patient with a lesion primarily in area 22 has profound difficulty with the interpretation of sounds; the spoken language may be utterly meaningless or extremely difficult to comprehend. *Expressive* (*motor*) *aphasia* is a disturbance in which thoughts are not expressed orally or in writing in a meaningful way. Lesions in the posterior temporoparietal region have been implicated. *Apraxia* is the inability to perform certain skilled and complex movements, even though there is no paralysis or disturbance in motor coordination and the sensory pathways are functioning normally. Lesions in the various cortical areas (supramarginal gyrus, other regions of the parietal and occipital lobes, premotor cortex, and Broca's speech areas 44 and 45), the association fibers interconnecting many of these cortical areas, and the corpus callosum may result in several types of apraxias. Among these are (1) the inability to perform skilled learned movements; this ranges from the clumsy execution of writing and drawing to *agraphia*, a condition in which the subject cannot write; (2) the inability to carry out a sequence of complex motor acts (often called *transmissive apraxia*); e.g., a subject who is able to brush his teeth, comb his hair, wash his face, and tie his shoes automatically is unable, upon command, to perform these tasks in that sequence (lesion in the supramarginal gyrus); and (3) the loss of articulate speech (often called *oral aphasia*) with otherwise normal musculature of the tongue, lips, larynx, and palate. The subject has use of only a few words in conversation and mispronounces common words or repeats the same word over and over again (lesion in Broca's areas 44 and 45 and in other regions).

"MOTOR AREAS"

Primary Motor Cortex

This cortex, often called the "motor cortex," is located in area 4 of the precentral gyrus (Figs. 20.3 and 22.4). Direct topical electric stimulation of this region evokes movements of the voluntary muscles. A map of this electrically excitable motor cortex produces the configuration of a homunculus, indicative of the somatotopic representation of different parts of the body. This homunculus is upside down, with the head region near the lateral fissure and with the lower extremity on the medial surface in the paracentral lobule. The amount of the motor cortex devoted to specific regions is roughly proportional to the delicacy of control of that region (e.g., large areas for fingers, thumb, lips, and tongue). The ablation of this "motor cortex" results in marked contralateral paresis, flaccidity, hyperactive deep tendon reflexes, and positive Babinski reflex, and is followed by moderate motor recovery. (Note similarities and differences to upper motor neuron paralysis; see Chap. 9.)

Premotor Cortex and Supplementary Motor Area (Fig. 22.4)

The premotor cortex consists of areas 6 and 8. On the medial aspect of the frontal lobe in area 6 is the supplementary motor area. Stimulation of this supplemental area elicits responses that outline a small homunculus with its head located rostrally. These responses are largely bilateral synergistic movements of tonic or postural nature, affecting primarily the axial muscles and proximal muscles of the extremities. Stimulation of area 6 on the lateral cerebral surface produces adversive movements—these "orientation" movements are generalized actions, such as turning of the head and eyes, twisting movements of the trunk, and general flexion or extension of the limbs. Stimulation of area 8, eye field, results in conjugate movements of the eyes to the opposite sides. This frontal eye field influences the volitional eye movements. Bilateral ablations of the supplementary motor area on the medial aspect of the frontal lobe in the rhesus monkey result in hypertonus of flexor muscles and increase in resistance to passive movements in the limbs, but no paresis. Symptoms of upper motor neuron paralysis are probably the result of interruption of fibers from the primary motor cortex, supplementary motor cortex, and premotor cortex. A second motor area coextensive with the secondary somatic sensory area has been described.

Prefrontal Cortex

The prefrontal cortex (areas 9 through 12) and its rich connections with the dorsomedial nucleus of the thalamus, hypothalamus, and limbic system are well developed in man. The prefrontal lobe has been conceived as being a regulator of the depth of feeling of an individual. It is not involved in the perception of sensations, but rather in the "affect" associated with the sensation. The complex responses of an individual, from calmness to ecstasy, from gloom to elation, from friendliness to disagreeableness, have their roots in areas 9 to 12. The bilateral ablation of areas of the prefrontal cortex or interruption of the subcortical white matter (*prefrontal lobotomy, leukotomy*) may produce subjects who are less excitable and less creative. Relief from anxiety is accompanied by a change in the patient's outlook and disposition. Drive, not intelligence, is altered. Relief from intractable pain is obtained. The pain remains, but the patient is unconcerned about it because the psychic feeling associated with the intensity of the pain is lost. A modern concept suggests that the prefrontal cortex is the neocortical representative of the limbic system.

"PSYCHICAL CORTEX"

The neocortex of the anterior pole of the temporal lobe has been called the "psychical cortex," because the responses obtained by electrical stimulation of this area include associations relative to "experiences." Stimulation may elicit the recall of objects seen or of music heard. Visual and auditory hallucinations may be produced, e.g., illusions which are similar to objects felt, seen, or heard in everyday experience. The illusion may be a clear reenactment, unencumbered by confusion, of an experience of the recent or distant past. The elicited experience may be a symphonic melody that the subject thinks is being played on a phonograph or on a radio. The patient with temporal lobe tumors may have auditory and visual hallucinations. He may see vivid scenes and friends not present and he may hear songs not being sung.

SPLIT-BRAIN MAN AND CEREBRAL DOMINANCE

The presence of several commissures in the cerebrum—including the corpus callosum with its 300 million fibers in humans—suggests that interhemispheric fiber pathways are of crucial significance to the functioning of the brain. Yet when the corpus callosum is completely transected, even in humans, no functional alterations can be detected by the usual neurologic and psychologic examinations. Complex activities, such as playing musical instruments and writing, are performed with the same dexterity as prior to sectioning of the corpus callosum.

An experimental animal or human being with a transected corpus callosum and other commissures (anterior and hippocampal commissures) has, in a way, two brains; such individuals are called *twin-brain* or *split-brain* people. They behave normally, are alert and curious, perceive, learn, and retain learned activities as do normal animals and human beings.

Studies of split-brain monkeys and human beings have been conducted so that the input from the periphery has been projected to only one hemisphere. The memories of perceptually learned information and of learned motor activities are apparently confined to the hemisphere to which the sensory information was relayed and from which the motor output was projected. If the corpus callosum is intact, this memory is utilized for motor expression by both hemispheres. Apparently the *engram,* or *memory trace,* laid down in the directly trained hemisphere is transferred via the callosal fibers to the opposite hemisphere, and a second engram is laid down in the contralateral hemisphere. The inference is that the corpus callosum transfers information from one hemisphere to the other. The corpus callosum may be utilized by the uneducated hemisphere to tap the engram of the trained hemisphere.

The left cerebral hemisphere is considered to be dominant over the right hemisphere in naturally right-handed individuals; the right hemisphere is dominant in naturally left-handed individuals. The phenomenon of *cerebral dominance* is known, but the degree to which it applies is not precisely understood. Dominance may reflect an asymmetry of morphologic and physiologic organization, and it may be an expression of unilateral engram formation. Apparently most cortical engrams are laid down bilaterally (double sets), or are formed unilaterally and readily transferred via callosal and anterior commissural fibers to the other hemisphere. In human beings, speech and the language symbolisms of the written and spoken word are lateralized in the dominant hemisphere. Both the dominant (or "talking") hemisphere and the nondominant ("mute") hemisphere can comprehend, but normally only the dominant hemisphere "talks." Linguistic expression resides exclusively within the dominant hemisphere, whereas the comprehension of both the written and spoken language is represented in both hemispheres.

Split-brain human subjects do exhibit some interesting and curious disabilities. The ultimate expression of the general sensory information which is conveyed from the right hand to the left or dominant hemisphere may differ dramatically from that which is conveyed from the left hand to the right or nondominant hemisphere. The right hand may be "unaware" of what the left hand is doing; for example, the right hand may be buttoning the patient's shirt while the left hand is unbuttoning it. The subject can name an object held in the right hand but cannot name an object held in the left hand; the act of naming is a function of the dominant hemisphere. Patients can perform certain tasks better with the left hand than with the right hand. This indicates that the nondominant hemisphere does have some superior roles over the dominant hemisphere. For example, better performances are executed by the left hand than by the right hand in tasks involving spatial relations such as arranging blocks, drawing simple three-dimensional objects (cubes), and matching up designs.

Roughly 90 percent of adults are right-handed. In these right-handers the left hemisphere is motor-dominant because the cerebral motor center on the left side controls the right hand. In left-handers, the right hemisphere is considered to be dominant for handedness. In about 98 percent of the adults, the comprehension of the spoken and written word as well as the motor control of language (speech) are expressions of the left cerebral hemisphere. Only in about 2 percent of the population are the speech centers (e.g., Broca's areas 44 and 45) located in the right hemisphere.

Apparently the lateralization of *speech centers* is not casually related to handedness. About 90 percent of right-handers have speech centers in the left hemisphere, while the other 10 percent have speech centers in the right hemisphere. About 65 percent of left-handers have speech centers in the left hemisphere, 20 percent in the right hemisphere, and the remaining 15 percent have speech centers located bilaterally. Naturally ambidextrous subjects have their speech centers located as follows: 60 percent in the left hemisphere, 10 percent in the right hemisphere, and 30 percent in both hemispheres. Stated otherwise, speech functions are lateralized to the left hemisphere in most adults, regardless of hand preference. Some individuals have speech centers located in the right hemisphere while a few others have speech centers in both hemispheres.

Index